YOUR VOICE, YOUR CHOICE

June 2017

YOUR VOICE, YOUR CHOICE

Personalizing Your Healthcare Decisions

To Jo and Arnold,
May peace be with you!
With love and thanks,
Catherine

Catherine Pesek Bird

Bird, Catherine Pesek
Your Voice, Your Choice: Personalizing Your Healthcare Decisions/ Catherine Pesek Bird. 1st edition
ISBN-13: 9780998661605
ISBN-10: 0998661600
Library of Congress Control Number: 2017904873
Dog & Bird Publishing, Chicago, Illinois

Production Credits
Cover design: Seania McCarthy
Internal Design: CreateSpace
Author photograph: John Reilly Photography

Dog & Bird Publishing
info@DogandBirdPublishing.com
Chicago, Illinois

Go confidently in the direction of your dreams. Live the life you have imagined.

—HENRY DAVID THOREAU

Catherine Pesek Bird is a physician, author, speaker, consultant, and certified medical mediator. She comes from a family of physicians and funeral home owners/morticians. As such, she has an appreciation for both helping to preserve life and helping to accept death, honoring the person's wishes in both situations. She has worked with many clients, helping them to personalize their healthcare decisions and to empower their agents to speak for them when their voices cannot be heard.

After earning her medical degree, Catherine completed a residency in internal medicine, in addition to a fellowship in cardiovascular diseases, and earned an MBA from the University of Notre Dame. She was a practicing cardiologist for several years. Currently, she resides in Chicago with her husband and children.

Contents

To everything there is a season, and a time for every purpose.

ECCLESIASTES 3:1

By failing to prepare, you are preparing to fail.

—Benjamin Franklin

More than twenty years ago, I graduated from medical school in Chicago. I can remember that the first time I was called "Doctor," I looked to see if the person was speaking to my father. I am most grateful to all my patients for entrusting their care to me. I have learned so much from them. The ones I remember best were those who realized when more could have been done *to* them but accepted that more should not have been done *for* them. Their courage continues to inspire me.

Health issues of my own eventually made seeing patients impossible for me. I tried to hold on to the satisfaction that practicing medicine and caring for patients gave me, including working on the administrative side of health care. However, at the end of the day, I found that I missed being directly involved in helping patients and their families.

A dear friend who is a very successful mediator recognized something in me and suggested I become a certified medical mediator. I followed her advice and completed the necessary coursework. In mediating medical issues, I often found myself trying to assist in contentious situations where patients were not able to speak for themselves, and various relatives were not in agreement on the best course of medical action.

After one particularly difficult session, one of the relatives involved in the fracas asked what I could do for him now so that *his* voice would be heard even if he could not speak. I worked with him and his spouse, helping them to determine what options they each would choose if they found themselves unable to have their voices heard.

We also identified who they wanted as agents or healthcare surrogates. Then we had a session where they explained their wishes to their agents not only so that the agents would hear their wishes but also so that they were fully involved in the conversation and could appreciate the context in which the decision was reached.

That was the start of my helping clients to personalize their advanced directives. More than once, I have been told that by empowering agents in this way, they can respond when called upon with much greater certainty that their responses are truly representative of what is wanted.

From there, I developed the materials that I am sharing with you in this book. My hope is that you will (1) read the book and see yourself in these pages, (2) identify your healthcare surrogate, proxy, or agent (whichever label works for you), and (3) share with that person exactly what your wishes are so that your voice will be heard even if you cannot speak.

How to Read This Book

In the case of good books, the point is not to see how many of them you can get through, but rather how many can get through to you.

—MORTIMER ADLER

Thank you for choosing this book. As you read through it, please see yourself and your loved ones in these pages. Read it as if I were in the room with you, helping to explain the various options. Although I am trained as a physician, I am not offering medical or legal advice in this book. I am simply explaining options that may or may not be offered to you during a hospital stay.

Take the time to discuss which of these options might work for you if you were in a situation where supportive treatment was offered. Then share those thoughts—why they might work or why you think they would not be best for you—with the people you trust the most: your spouse, your adult children, your bridge partner, or your friend down the hall. It doesn't matter with whom you share your choices; just make certain that you do.

But for this to work, you must not only discuss it but also make certain your choices are documented. In most cases, that means completing a durable power of attorney for healthcare decisions form. This form is available in all fifty states, although it may differ in format. If you are a veteran receiving care through the US Department of Veterans Affairs (VA), it has its own version, which is valid throughout the VA system.

If you reside in multiple states, then consider using the form that is accepted in your legal state of residence. Check with your attorney for advice on this. In fact, as you are completing the form, I encourage you to discuss any questions that arise with your healthcare providers and your attorney as well as any other professionals who are assisting you with your affairs.

After the form is completed, some states require it to be witnessed, some states require it to be notarized, and some states require it to be both witnessed and notarized. When you have completed all the requirements, consider providing a copy for your physicians, your attorney, your agent, and any others you think should be aware. Only your designated agent will be called upon to answer any questions from the physicians caring for you, but informing other loved ones of your wishes can make for smoother acceptance on their part. Additionally, be certain to bring a copy with you when you visit any physician, hospital, or clinic.

Now, let's get started, shall we?

Section 1: How We Got Here

Those who cannot remember the past are condemned to repeat it.

—George Santayana

I tend to drone on to my children about historic facts that are absolutely fascinating to me. My children, amazingly to me, do not always find my stories anywhere near as fascinating as I do, but they are kind enough to listen. Had I not become a physician, I would have been a history professor.

I share this with you because, in this chapter, I could be accused of droning on a bit. It is my nature. Please bear with me. When discussing any new topic, I have always been drawn to learning its history. By understanding its origins, I know that I can then make better sense of the topic. My hope is that this section will help you in this way also.

How did we get to the point of having these choices? What life-sustaining, or organ-sustaining, medical treatments are there, and when might we need to accept them? My answer is to look at the history of three areas:

1. The development of new medical technologies
2. The landmark cases in medical decision making
3. The role of advanced directives

Development of New Medical Technologies

Cure sometimes, treat often, comfort always.

—HIPPOCRATES

HOW TECHNOLOGY IMPACTS LIVES

My father was a pioneer cardiothoracic surgeon. He and his team developed the first heart-lung bypass machine in Chicago. They used the machine to repair a severe congenital heart defect that a young child had since birth.

Without the surgery, the child would not have survived to adulthood. Without the heart-lung bypass machine, the surgery would have been impossible. By replacing the work of the heart and lungs with this machine, this young child's heart could be stopped and the surgery performed. After all the stitches were in place, they could restart the heart and remove the machine. The child survived, thrived, and went on to have a family of his own.

SUCCESS BUILDS ON SUCCESS

This surgery occurred in the 1950s. The ability to successfully perform groundbreaking surgery depends not only upon new technologies but also upon prior medical discoveries. Without these pioneers in medicine, we would not have the array of choices that we have today. And today's inventions will be tested and modified to become tomorrow's standard of care.

CARDIAC ARREST

The specific technologies that I would like us to focus on here are those commonly considered in a cardiac-arrest situation. That is when someone is not breathing and without a pulse. These advances are the cornerstone of current therapy.

IT ALL STARTS WITH A, B, C

When teaching a class, in responding to a person who is "found down," we teach students to follow their ABCs. First, look for A, an airway, to make certain the person is not choking. If the airway is not obstructed, then we ask the students to move on to B and check for breathing, or spontaneous respirations. Then we move on to C, for circulation, which requires looking for a pulse. These are the basic signs of life that everyone taking a first aid class learns. It is also a good idea to call for help, as in activating Emergency Medical Services (EMS), which in most communities can be accomplished by dialing 911.

SO THAT THE LUNGS MAY RISE AND TAKE AIR

The idea that both an airway and breathing are important for life is not a new concept. We can look all the way back to the second century, when a physician by the name of Galen noted the importance of breathing, or ventilation, to maintain life. Unfortunately, the brilliance of his ideas was lost to the world for a long period of time.

After the world got though the (truly) Dark Ages, fortunately another scientist, Andreas Vesalius, learned about Galen's ideas and expanded on his work on the importance of breathing. The year was 1543; it marks the start of the Scientific Revolution, or the *annus mirabilis*, the miracle year. At that time, Vesalius wrote in *De humani corporis fabrica libri septum*:

But that life may be restored to the animal, an opening must be attempted into the trunk of the trachea, into which a tube of reed or cane should be put; you will blow into this, so that the lungs may rise again and take air.

Unfortunately, this simple but stunningly brilliant concept of placing a tube into the trachea (the connection in the throat between the mouth and the lungs) was lost until the 1700s. During this time, other, less direct methods of artificial respiration were tried, including rolling the patient over a barrel. As you can imagine, varying degrees of success were achieved with such techniques.

So, we learned that breathing into the mouth could blow air into the lungs. The idea of mouth-to-mouth respiration was first used in the 1740s to help drowning victims who were rescued from the Seine River in Paris. Later, in the 1950s, we determined that the exhaled breath from one person could be blown effectively into another person's mouth. This would provide enough air, without the need for bellows (a household device squeezed to deliver air and thereby increase the flames in a fire) or a barrel.

THE IRON LUNG AND OTHER VENTILATORS
Even with the success of mouth-to-mouth respiration, devices to force air from outside the body persisted, and body-enclosing devices were developed. One type was known as the iron lung. It was used extensively for polio victims who, due to severe respiratory muscle involvement, were unable to breath on their own.

A BLAST FROM THE PAST
In the 1950s, it was noted that many polio patients with respiratory muscle paralysis were dying despite iron lung therapy. Bjorn Ibsen, a physician in Boston, recommended replacing the body-enclosing device with a familiar idea from a few hundred years

prior: place a tube directly into the patient's trachea, and blow air into the tube.

GOODBYE, IRON LUNG, HELLO, DIRECT INTUBATION

Patients were removed from body-enclosing devices and directly intubated, which means having a tube placed from the lips down the throat and into the trachea. The mortality rate from respiratory failure due to polio decreased overnight. However, as there was no automated way to blow air into the tracheal tube, it had to be done manually.

THE BIRTH OF THE INTENSIVE CARE UNIT

Due to the intensity of care required to have someone assigned to literally squeeze air into a tube around the clock, patients who required this degree of specialized care were all moved to one area of the hospital, hence the birth of the intensive care unit (ICU). Fortunately, automatic mechanical ventilators soon followed, so the medical staff could get on with other duties, but the ICU lives on.

Now ICUs are even more specialized. In many larger hospitals, there could be a pediatric ICU, a medical ICU, a surgical ICU, and perhaps even a neurosurgical ICU and a cardiovascular ICU. Specific needs of patients can be better addressed by centralizing the required resources in terms of nursing expertise, equipment, and physicians.

CARDIOPULMONARY RESUSCITATION AND DEFIBRILLATION

We've covered the A and the B, or the airway and breathing parts of the problem. Now let's move on to the system near and dear to my heart (excuse the pun), the circulatory system. By searching for a pulse in a person's arms, legs, or neck, we are determining whether the heart is pumping. By checking the rate and rhythm of the pulse, we are determining whether the pumping is considered effective.

WHAT TO DO IF THERE'S NO PULSE

In 1903, the first successful use of external chest compressions, or pushing on the chest from the outside to mimic the pumping of the heart, was reported. Cardiopulmonary resuscitation (CPR) brought together mouth-to-mouth respiration treatment with external chest compressions as a therapy for patients found to be unresponsive. In 1960, training programs in CPR and defibrillation were developed and taught by the American Heart Association, first for physicians and later for laypeople, as a treatment for unresponsive patients.

BRIDGE TO SUCCESS

Today, CPR is a temporary means to maintain some degree of blood flow and oxygenation for a person who is not breathing and has no pulse. It is a bridge to more definitive treatment for the return to normal cardiac rhythm and breathing.

CPR relies on (1) pressing down on the patient's chest to literally make the heart squeeze at a rapid rate, thereby allowing blood to flow throughout the body, and (2) supplying the lungs with oxygen by breathing into the patient's opened mouth.

This is important, because the body, including the brain, depends on blood to bring oxygen to the cells. Without oxygenated blood flowing, a person at normal room temperature would experience brain damage in just a few minutes. The goal of CPR, then, is to maintain oxygenated blood flow throughout the body.

After an extended period, anyone performing CPR needs to be relieved, as it is a physically intense procedure. And CPR alone does not usually allow for a poorly beating heart to function well enough for a person to return to normal heart rhythm without further intervention.

To restore normal cardiac rhythm, we should think of the heart as what it is, a muscle. It is a very important and highly specialized muscle, but it is a muscle all the same. As a muscle, it contracts and relaxes.

You can control the muscles in your arms and legs so that they move. By contracting and relaxing muscles, we control movement. Some muscles move voluntarily or only when we think about moving them. The heart, luckily for us, does not contract only when we think about it.

The heart is made up of a special type of muscle found only in the heart, simply called cardiac muscle. Normally, the heart contracts and relaxes, or beats. A special area within the heart that sends out electrical signals regulates this beating. Keep that electrical thought for just a moment, and let's look at this further.

CARDIAC DEFIBRILLATION

Back in 1849, in the early days of the California gold rush, it was discovered that using too much chloroform as an anesthetic during surgery could cause a beating heart to stop. To remedy this situation when it arose, surgeons would stop the operation and move their attention to the patient's chest, and if the inside of the chest was not already easily accessible, then they would proceed by making a rather large incision across the chest and manually squeeze the heart, known as direct or open-cardiac massage.

Fortunately, in 1958, it was noted that applying an electric current through a defibrillator directly to the chest wall could achieve the same effect without requiring the surgeon's hands to literally be inside the chest and around the heart. I feel confident in saying that the postoperative infection rate and the surgical survival rate both likely benefitted from this new approach.

AUTOMATIC EXTERNAL DEFIBRILLATORS

As technology of defibrillators improved, the automatic external defibrillator (AED) was introduced. The AED has built-in algorithmic logic, so trained bystanders, who are not medical personnel, only need to attach the leads as illustrated on the machine and then get out of the way. These devices were adopted for public-access defibrillation and have been used successfully in airports, shopping centers, office buildings, and even on international flights.

PRESSOR AGENTS

So, now we have discussed how we can artificially promote breathing and heart beating, or circulation. This is important to maintain blood flow through the heart and to the brain. However, other organs also need good blood flow to maintain function.

In the hierarchy of organ function, think of the brain, the heart, and the lungs as the "big three," which we will discuss in detail a bit later. I recall a colleague who is a pulmonologist (a lung doctor). He used to joke with me, the cardiologist, that the lungs were the two big organs that had to be working to keep the little organ, the heart, going. Then another friend, a neurosurgeon (brain surgeon), would come by and remind us that the function of the lungs and the heart didn't really matter if the brain wasn't working. He got the last word then and still does now.

Once we are secure in the knowledge that we are helping the brain to get oxygen, thanks to the lungs and the heart, then the next organ system we want to focus attention on is the kidneys, as they are the filtration system for the body. Without adequate blood flow to the kidneys, they will stop working, and then you have a lot of problems. When looking at a patient, physicians look at what organ systems are not working, and once you get beyond two organ systems failing, the patient's ability to recover becomes more remote, as in not very likely.

In other words, if your lungs are working only because of the ventilator and you have another organ system or more fail, then the odds that you will walk out of the hospital are not good.

To help maintain adequate blood pressure, some very strong medicines can be given that selectively allow blood to flow to vital areas such as the kidneys. These medicines are collectively known as pressor agents, from the French word *presser*, meaning "to squeeze." Think of these pressor agents as selectively making the heart beat stronger. These agents are not without complications and are usually only given in the ICU for as short a period as needed.

I know this is a lot to digest, but I wanted you to have a perspective on the basics of what is important and why when a person is found down. Having a loved one in the ICU can be overwhelming. It can be daunting just seeing the person in the bed, sometimes looking small and weak, surrounded by so much medical equipment. Hopefully this section will have provided you with some idea of what can be done when caring for a seriously ill patient either in a cardiac arrest situation or in the ICU.

SUMMARY

- Medical advances have provided us with a way to attempt to artificially support life for someone who is found down.
- CPR is a way to provide respiratory and circulatory support, but it is a bridge. Most patients are not going to recover with just CPR.
- Intubation and mechanical ventilation can help support the lungs to function.
- Cardiac defibrillation is the delivery of an electric shock to the chest with the intent to return the heart to a perfusable rhythm, which means it effectively delivers oxygenated blood to the brain and other parts of the body.
- The AED is a great invention that provides early access to a means of effectively returning the heart to a perfusable rhythm.
- Pressor agents are very strong medications that can help support blood flow to the kidneys (and other organs) so that they continue to function.

Landmark Cases of Medical Decision Making

We can rebuild him. We have the technology.

FROM *The Six Million Dollar Man*

SETTING THE LANDSCAPE

In the last chapter, we reviewed medical inventions and interventions that allow physicians to keep patients alive. We discussed keeping a heart beating by chest compressions and electrical intervention and keeping the lungs working by mechanical ventilation. We also discussed how medications such as pressor agents can help to maintain blood flow to preserve kidney function.

Due to these interventions, some would say that we can maintain life. However, the quality of that life is sometimes deemed unacceptable, especially if the person is not aware of his or her surroundings. Often, because of a prolonged period without adequate oxygenation to the brain prior to the introduction of these interventions, there can be a degree of brain damage. The damage may be such that the person's level of awareness is not expected to improve. This is usually the time when a decision needs to be made whether to continue with the treatment or not.

With this potential disconnect between what can be done *to* a patient and what can be done *for* a patient, there can be conflict among the patient's family members, caregivers, and care facilities. Some select cases have set the tone for how these conflicts are resolved. I would like to discuss a few of these with you.

ENDURING THE UNENDURABLE

On April 14, 1975, a twenty-one-year-old woman ingested many tranquilizer pills. She then went to a bar and drank several alcoholic beverages. While at the bar, she passed out, never to regain consciousness.

She was taken back to her residence by a housemate. During this time, she had at least two episodes where she was not breathing, each episode lasting at least fifteen minutes. The housemate administered mouth-to-mouth resuscitation and called for an ambulance. In the ambulance, she received supplemental oxygen by face mask.

Early in the morning of April 15, 1975, she was admitted to a local hospital and was intubated and ventilated with the assistance of a mechanical respirator. She was later transferred to another hospital for a higher level of care. Over the next few months, she remained in a state of unconsciousness, called a persistent vegetative state, which was attributed to the prolonged lack of oxygen and resulting brain damage. She underwent a tracheostomy, replacing the tube down her throat for a tube that enters her body through a small incision in her neck, which allowed the mechanical ventilator to continue assisting her ability to breathe, without the tube pressing and causing damage to her throat.

Her weight had been one hundred fifteen pounds on admission to the hospital. After a few months, she was down to less than seventy pounds. Examinations revealed irreversible brain damage.

Her next of kin were her parents. The physicians shared with them the fact that there was no prospect of recovery for their daughter. The parents then asked that she be removed from the ventilator. The attending physicians on the case refused to do so, despite the parents signing a statement waiving any potential liability from removing the ventilator.

In coming to this decision, the parents had sought counsel from their Roman Catholic priest. The priest, in providing counseling, quoted Pope Pius XII's declaration from 1957 that "there is no moral obligation to continue extraordinary means to sustain life when there is no realistic hope of recovery." Thus, the parents went to court, petitioning that their daughter be allowed to die.

After a lower court's decision that removal of the respirator could not be allowed, as it could violate the state's homicide statutes, the parents took the case to the New Jersey Supreme Court. On March 31, 1976, the court unanimously agreed with the parents. In the court's opinion, "no compelling interest of the state could compel [one] to endure the unendurable, only to vegetate a few measurable months with no realistic possibility of returning to any semblance of cognitive or sapient state."

The patient was weaned from the ventilator and transferred to a nursing home. She survived more than ten years from that initial night. Under the direction of her parents, no further extraordinary measures were taken, other than maintaining food and water through a feeding tube. The end came on June 11, 1985; she died from pneumonia.

MINIMALLY CONSCIOUS

In another part of the country, a twenty-six-year-old woman was at home in the early hours of February 25, 1990, when her heart stopped functioning properly, and she fell to the ground. Her husband called for emergency medical services.

Upon the paramedics' arrival, she was found to be in full cardiac arrest, requiring multiple attempts of electric shocks to successfully defibrillate her heart to a perfusable rhythm. She was transferred to a local hospital for further care.

After admission to the hospital, testing was done to try to determine the cause of her cardiac arrest. It was noted that her blood level of the essential electrolyte sodium was low, which was attributed as the cause of her cardiac arrest. This imbalance was easily treated and corrected.

However, the amount of downtime, the period when her heart was not pumping adequately to perfuse her brain and the rest of her body with oxygenated blood, caused severe brain damage. She remained in a coma for three months.

She then became somewhat aware of her surroundings and did not require mechanical ventilation for respiratory support; she could breathe unaided. After several examinations by various experts in the field of neurology (the study of the function of the brain and the nervous system), it was determined that she was in either a persistent vegetative state or a minimally conscious state.

She was transferred to another care facility. A feeding tube supported her nutritional needs. The tube entered her body through an incision in the skin over her abdomen and was advanced into her stomach.

In this case, the debate was between her husband and her parents as to whether or not she would want to live in this state. Her husband argued that she had previously stated that she would not want to live attached to tubes. Her parents argued that the feeding tube should not be removed.

The debate took many years to be resolved in the court system. This also played out for the public by the media and politicians.

In the end, over a decade and a half after her collapse, her husband's request was honored. Against her parents' wishes, the feeding tube was removed. Thirteen days later, on March 31, 2005, she died.

She was forty-one years old.

BRAIN DEAD BUT PREGNANT

On November 26, 2013, in the wee hours of the morning on the Tuesday before Thanksgiving, a thirty-three-year-old paramedic and mother went into the kitchen of her Texas home to prepare a bottle for her toddler. It was the last thing she willfully did. She then collapsed to the floor and was down for an unknown time, with some estimates that she was down for at least one hour. Her husband, who was also a paramedic, found her down. He performed CPR on his wife until the on-duty team arrived.

She was transferred to a local hospital, and medical treatments were done to stabilize her: she was intubated and attached to a mechanical ventilator. Studies showed that the cause of her cardiac arrest was likely a pulmonary embolism, a blood clot that may have traveled from her leg to her lung, blocking the lung's ability to function and oxygenate her blood. Additionally, studies showed that she was brain dead, with total loss of all higher brain function.

As a paramedic, she had verbally made it known to her husband and family members that she did not want to be on a ventilator if there was no hope for her recovery. The family shared this information with the hospital. They then gathered for what they thought would be the honoring of these wishes by termination of the mechanical ventilation.

However, the hospital informed the family that, due to Texas law, as she was fourteen weeks pregnant, her wishes could not be honored. She would have to stay on the mechanical ventilation until she delivered the fetus. This was despite studies showing that the child would not be viable, as it had also been deprived of oxygen for an extended period.

The family turned to the court system to plead their case. The courts agreed that the patient was brain dead, and as such, Texas state law did not apply to her. The hospital was ordered to declare the patient dead. No appeal was filed, and on January 26, 2014, the ventilator was removed, and the patient was declared legally dead.

NO VOICE, WHAT CHOICE?

I bring up these three cases for your review. It is not my intent to argue the law; I am not an attorney. I am not attempting to make a case in any way for or against the medical treatments provided. Although I am a licensed physician, I was never involved in the care of any of these patients. I have not written this book to give medical or legal advice. Nor do I wish to debate the ethics or motives for what decisions were made.

My reason for mentioning these cases is to illustrate for you what can happen when people are no longer able to speak for themselves. I bring up these real-life dramas because they played out in the public eye. Although we have no way of knowing, I doubt that any of these people wanted the fame from the debates that will forever be associated with their deaths.

In writing these cases, I purposefully have not used their names or any specific details other than those I feel are necessary to make my points.

SUMMARY

The main point is this: if you want to have a voice in what happens to you, if you are not able to speak for yourself, then you need to act now.

Next, we will review how that can be achieved.

3

Advanced Directives: Make Your Wishes Known

Death, a necessary end, will come when it will come.

—William Shakespeare, *Julius Caesar*

SPEAK NOW, OR FOREVER HOLD YOUR PEACE

In the last chapter, we reviewed three cases that illustrate how, in modern times, our advances in medical technology can cause conflicts with perceived wishes. In all three cases:

- They were relatively young people.
- They were without known medical issues that we would identify as terminal illnesses.
- They were not expecting to be in the situation that resulted.

Yet they went, literally overnight, from a normal state of health to a state in which they were never going to be able to speak for themselves again. They were not prepared, nor were their loved ones or healthcare providers.

The family members in each case commented on what they believed the patient's wishes were. Yet none of these patients were known to have written any form of advanced directive to cover any medical issues that might arise. Without a written form of their wishes, it was left up to the courts to determine the best course of action involving their lives.

HOW WILL YOU BE REMEMBERED?

I don't think any of us would want to pit one family member against another or to have our family members arguing our case in either a hospital or care facility or in a courtroom. Yet so few of us take any action before it is too late. This isn't golf; there are no do-overs or mulligans. I make a joke here not to be cruel but to illustrate my point. I realize that this is not an easy topic; sometimes life is hard. Without addressing the way you want these things handled, you are not preparing yourself or your loved ones. And you may end up with no one knowing what you really want.

I truly would like for you to be prepared. I am assuming, since you are reading this, that you would like that too, for yourself and your loved ones. Let's take a deeper dive into what we can learn from these cases. And let's look at how we can be prepared— how can we avoid becoming a topic of debate within our families, among our healthcare providers, or with the legal system.

MEANINGFUL RECOVERY

To me, the three patients and their stories help us to define *meaningful recovery*. In all three cases, the patients were functional, and then something happened that left them with an altered level of consciousness and awareness. Additionally, all three patients required some level of invasive medical technology, whether it was mechanical ventilation or a feeding tube, to maintain them.

The first case truly was the sentinel case to look at how advances in medical technology such as mechanical ventilation could be utilized. Although the patient was young and had no known underlying medical conditions, the amount of time without oxygen severely altered her ability to interact with the world as we know it.

Her parents also were distressed at what they perceived as her "fighting" or "bucking" the ventilator. In the 1970s, ventilator settings were not as advanced as they are now, and it was more difficult to adjust them. This perception of pain from the ventilator seems to have contributed to the parents wanting its removal.

But the overarching issue from these cases, in my opinion, is that we need to carefully consider when continuing with invasive medical care, such as mechanical ventilation, results in improved outcomes versus when the patient is done, with no hope for return to a cognitive state. These cases opened the door for more legislation to allow patients to define their desires in terms of invasive medical technology. It helped to spark interest in people speaking for themselves, while they still can, in terms of a living will.

In the first case, we had family members at odds with what they saw as the right thing to do for a patient. This unfortunately occurs with some frequency. From a legal perspective, a legal next of kin will be identified or a court-appointed guardian may be named, but someone will have the last word on what happens.

The family members in the second case had very different opinions on what they thought was best for the patient. The patient's wishes were not written and were not clearly detailed. The courts ultimately sided with the husband; he was the legal next of kin.

In the last case, the patient's wishes were well known. Her husband and her parents agreed on what her wishes were and how they wanted those wishes honored. However, an interpretation of a state law caused the healthcare facility to have a different opinion of what could be done. Special circumstances, such as pregnancy, minority age, and competency, must also be considered.

HAVING YOUR SAY

These cases could be viewed as a call to action to address these issues before we cannot speak for ourselves. But to help ensure that our wishes are honored, we must act. There are several documents that can assist in memorializing our wishes; collectively, they are referred to as advanced directives. Let's review the options so you can determine what might be appropriate for you:

- Orders for life-sustaining treatment (POLST, MOLST, or MOST)
- Do not resuscitate (DNR)
- Do not intubate (DNI)
- Living will
- Durable power of attorney for health care (DPOA-HC)

ORDER FOR LIFE-SUSTAINING TREATMENT

The order for life-sustaining treatment option is relatively new in terms of available advanced directives. It has various acronyms, depending on the exact name of the form used in various states. Examples include physician orders for life-sustaining treatment (POLST), medical orders for life-sustaining treatment (MOLST), and medical orders for scope of treatment (MOST). These are portable, physician-generated orders, usually reserved for terminally ill patients who may not want any of the life-sustaining treatments that we discussed in chapter 2.

Perhaps you recall hearing about emergency responders requested to come to the aid of a person at her residence, but the person had a known terminal illness and had already determined with her physician that she did not want life-sustaining treatments. Once the request for emergency medical services is made, though, the responding paramedics are obligated to treat the patient. Often, this results in treatment that does not honor the patient's wishes.

In the 1990s, a group in Oregon developed a process for how such patients' wishes could be honored, even when the patient was not physically in an acute care facility. This program spread to other states, with some subtle differences. The underlying process, though, is this: it is a portable order that reflects the patient's wishes, is sanctioned by the patient's treating physician, and allows the paramedics to withhold treatment as directed by the order, which can be personalized at the time it is written.

Although not a federal program, there is a national center that helps to standardize the various state programs. A goal of the program is that the patient's wishes can be recognized, even across state lines, if the patient travels to a state that also recognizes this process.

The process starts with a conversation between the patient and her healthcare provider that includes an understanding of the patient's diagnosis, prognosis, and possible treatment options, all in the context of the patient's goals for care, given her beliefs and values. The result of this conversation is an informed shared decision about the patient's choices of treatment in the event of a medical emergency.

The order is then printed on a bright piece of paper and signed by the physician; in some states, the patient also signs it. The bright piece of paper with the signed order should then be placed on the refrigerator door at a private residence or on the front of the patient's chart if in a care facility. If emergency personnel are called for the patient, then they can refer to the specifics noted in the POLST to guide their actions.

There has been some controversy regarding this process. The Catholic Church originally had concerns regarding the intention of this process. However, the POLST process does not allow for active euthanasia or physician-assisted suicide, as outlined in the 2009 edition of the *Ethical and Religious Directives for Catholic Health Care Services* authored by the United States Conference of Catholic Bishops.

Other key assumptions of this process must include (1) that the ordering physician truly understands the patient's beliefs and wishes, (2) that the patient truly understands the disease prognosis and treatment options, and (3) that the order can be rescinded, or voided, by the patient at any time.

Physicians and terminally ill patients in Oregon first developed the idea of a written order that would apply outside of the hospital. In this way, the order to withhold treatment, such as defibrillation and intubation, could be portable and follow the patient from an acute care facility to a long-term care facility to a private residence.

In some states, the process can be applied to patients who are minors and to patients with mental disabilities, with the consent of their guardians. The order can be rescinded and voided at any time.

DNR/DNI

Orders such as do not resuscitate (DNR) and do not intubate (DNI) are used in most states. They are also sometimes referred to as allow natural death (AND). This is an order, written by a physician, that is valid while you are hospitalized. The order directs healthcare providers not to resuscitate you. This kind of order is usually discussed during a hospital stay when a terminal illness has been identified and after you have the opportunity to understand your options.

This is like the POLST process; however, a key difference is that it is usually limited to only the current hospitalization during which it is written. It is usually not portable; it does not remain valid after discharge from the hospital or upon readmission.

The DNR order is often written when the patient states that he or she realizes CPR is often not successful, even when performed in a hospital, and can be very traumatic, since the chest compressions require a healthcare provider to push down directly on the patient's chest with both hands. The DNR clarifies that the patient does not want chest compressions or cardiac defibrillation (the application of electric shocks) to attempt to return the heart to a perfusable rhythm.

In some cases, a DNI is written instead of a DNR order. This allows for the resuscitation of CPR, cardiac defibrillation, and the use of medications such as pressor agents, but it prohibits intubation and mechanical ventilation. In the case of either a DNR or DNI order, comfort care, such as pain medication, is provided.

One of the limitations of this type of order is that it presumes you will be able to articulate your wishes throughout the hospital stay. If not, then you may not be able to articulate it if you change your mind on what you want done. And if for whatever reason you did not want a DNR/DNI order upon admission, then you would not be able to add one if your medical condition changed during that stay and you are unable to speak for yourself.

I mention this because a recent study showed that almost 80 percent of us, at some point during a hospital stay, may not be able to provide consent for ourselves. This may be due to the illness that necessitated our hospital stay, a complication that arose during the hospital stay, or the sedating effects of medications that may be required. When you consider only ICU patients, that number jumps to 95 percent of patients who, at some point in their hospital stay, are not able to provide consent for themselves.

LIVING WILL

A living will is a legally binding document that can be created and shared with your healthcare providers and loved ones. In it, you outline your goals of care and your wishes for what should be done for you in various medical scenarios. It is used if you are not able to speak for yourself. One limitation of a living will is that it can only cover what is listed within it.

DURABLE POWER OF ATTORNEY FOR HEALTH CARE

A durable power of attorney for health care decision form is also a legally binding document. It is very similar in nature to a power of attorney, which allows you to name an agent who is authorized to handle your financial affairs if you are incapacitated.

In the same way, a durable power of attorney allows you to name a healthcare agent, or proxy, who would speak for you regarding your medical issues if you were not able to speak for yourself. That agent would be authorized to speak to healthcare providers regarding your medical condition and prognosis. The agent would be empowered to authorize or refuse medical treatment.

This is extremely helpful when a person has no close family. A legal next of kin can be appointed by the state to speak for the patient, but that person may not be who the patient would truly want to speak for him or her. This assures that the agent is someone the patient trusts and wants in this role.

Naming a healthcare agent is also helpful when there is a large family. The hospital will determine the next of kin as defined by the state in which the patient is hospitalized. However, in a large family, there might be conflicting views held by various family members on what the patient would want if he or she could specify his or her choices. By naming an agent ahead of time, the person you want to speak for you will be authorized to do so.

Preplanning is needed when naming a healthcare agent. In order for this to work best, you need to be certain that the person you want as your agent feels that he or she can accomplish the task. And then you need to empower the person. You need to share your medical condition, your values, and your treatment goals. In this way, that person will truly be able to speak for you even when your voice cannot be heard.

Additionally, if there are people in your life whom you do not wish to be authorized to speak on your behalf, then you can add their names to the durable power of attorney document, effectively blocking their ability to make decisions on your behalf.

SUMMARY

- Eighty to 90 percent of patients, during some or all of their hospital stay, will not be able to speak for themselves.

- Advanced directives are just that, directives or orders that are completed in advance, while the person can give informed consent for what is done or not done to him or her.
- There are different advanced directives that may or may not be appropriate depending on the patient's medical condition.
- Orders for life-sustaining treatment might be an appropriate option for a patient with a terminal illness who has discussed with his or her physician his or her treatment goals and values.
- The portability of this type of order allows the patient's wishes to guide emergency medical services, first responders, paramedics, and emergency treatment center providers.
- DNR/DNI orders direct healthcare providers as to what a patient does and does not want done.
- Typically, these orders are only valid during a hospital stay; they usually do not transfer with the patient upon discharge to home or transfer to a long-term care facility.
- A living will allows you to write your treatment goals and values in a legally binding document that can be used by your healthcare providers to direct your care.
- Appointing a durable power of attorney for healthcare decisions allows you to name as your healthcare agent the person you really want to have speaking for you, whether it is your best friend, your spouse, or your bridge partner.
- For the greatest success in having your wishes followed, you need to empower your healthcare agent so that your voice will be heard even when you cannot speak.
- Please consult with your healthcare provider and your attorney to determine what options are best for you.

Section 2: What Choices We May Have

Knowing is not enough; we must apply. Willing is not enough; we must do.

—Johann Wolfgang von Goethe

APPLY AND DO

When I was in high school, my widowed grandfather and my widowed uncle moved in with my family. My father, the surgeon, suggested that my mother and I learn CPR. She and I went to classes taught at the local fire station and became certified. I never had to perform CPR on either my grandfather or my uncle.

However, during a huge snowstorm the day after Christmas when I was a senior in college, my mother collapsed next to the tree in our living room. As I had just been recertified in CPR, I immediately called for help and provided respiratory and circulatory support until the paramedics arrived. Despite my efforts and the efforts of the paramedics and the healthcare providers in the emergency department at the receiving hospital, my mother remained first comatose and then in a persistent vegetative state.

She was eventually weaned from the ventilator. Her care required a prolonged stay in a long-term care facility, then she "graduated" to a rehabilitation center. She eventually returned home. For the rest of her life, she required around-the-clock nursing care and a feeding tube to support her nutritionally.

TO WHAT END?

A few years later, she aspirated and developed pneumonia. She was suddenly very acutely ill on top of her chronic condition. I recall a conversation I, a young medical student at the time, had with my father regarding next steps.

He agreed with me that she could be hospitalized, given intravenous medicine to help her immune system fight the pneumonia, and undergo intubation and mechanical ventilation to take away the work of breathing while her body fought the infection. She might even require pressor agents if her blood pressure dropped to try to preserve her kidney function. He agreed that all this could be done to my mother, his wife.

But then he said something so profound, it stunned me. He asked me to what end that would bring us. Would treating her with antibiotics or pressor agents bring back the essence of what was my mother? Or had we already lost her on that snowy day many Decembers prior?

As my father so eloquently stated, at this point, it was not a question of what we could do *to* her. The important question was what could we do *for* her.

SUMMARY

- As you read these next chapters, please keep in mind what you would like to have done *to* you and what you would like to have done *for* you.
- Then please write down which options work for you under what circumstances. Share those with your chosen trusted agent.
- In this way, your choices will be known, and your voice will be heard.

4

Brain, Heart, and Lungs: The Big Three

If you think you can do a thing or think you can't do a thing, you're right.

—HENRY FORD

TO TUBE OR NOT TO TUBE

A true Southern gentleman had lung disease, the result of chemical exposure earlier in his life. A few of his friends had also developed this illness; therefore, he had a very clear understanding of what he was facing. His biggest concern was that his lung function would deteriorate, and he would need to live on a ventilator, which was something he did not think he could do. He shared this thinking with any healthcare provider he encountered. "Hello, my name is John, and I never want to be intubated," he would say.

One day, he did not feel well. His wife and daughter accompanied him to the emergency room (ER) of their community hospital. Although he did have this underlying lung problem, he had been doing rather well on supplemental oxygen at home. Up to this time, his lung disease had not required him to make many ER visits or to have many hospital stays. This day was different. He really was struggling to breathe, even at rest, despite supplemental oxygen. In the ER, the physicians examined him and performed the necessary tests to understand what was happening. They approached the bedside and told John, in front of his wife and daughter, that he had a bad lung infection and needed to be admitted to the hospital for intravenous (given through a vein) antibiotic treatment. Additionally, as the infection was so severe, they needed to take away the work of breathing by intubating and mechanically ventilating him for the next three days, after which they would reevaluate how he was doing.

His wife and daughter were shocked to hear this news; they told the physicians that John never wanted to be intubated. However, no one had ever discussed this concept of intubation and mechanical ventilation as a bridging therapy to help his lungs recover. The physicians explained to John and his family that they did not think this was a terminal event. They believed that John could recover if he was intubated and given antibiotics.

His wife and daughter were very hesitant to give consent for the intubation, knowing John's strong views against it. Additionally, they were not familiar with the idea of introducing intubation for a short period of time as a bridging therapy. The ER physicians were not his usual physicians but were virtual strangers to them. The family was not certain of the outcome if he were to start on this path of intubation. It was so different from what John had always told them. They were not certain what to say on his behalf.

Fortunately, John heard the discussion, and with his last bit of energy, he lifted a finger to get their attention. The physicians and the family bent down, trying to hear his words over the noise of the non-rebreather face mask that was providing him with high amounts of oxygen. They almost did not believe what they heard. John croaked, in a raspy voice, "Tube me!"

They proceeded immediately. Three days later, John's lung function was greatly improved. They weaned him off the ventilator, and he was discharged from the hospital.

After that, John changed his tune. "Tube me, if it will help," he said from then on. John survived a good four years after that event, which allowed him to attend his daughter's wedding.

THE BIG THREE, AND I DON'T MEAN FORD, GENERAL MOTORS, AND FIAT CHRYSLER

As we discussed before, the most important organs to maintain life as we know it are the brain, the heart, and the lungs. These are the big three! The body needs oxygenated blood to the brain and the heart via the lungs to maintain life. How well preserved the function of these three organ systems is determines how likely a person is to recover and walk out of the hospital.

THE BRAIN AND PREVENTING BRAIN DAMAGE

When a person's heart stops pumping, the brain is literally starved of oxygen. After three minutes at normal temperature, such as room temperature, this lack of oxygen can cause the brain to be damaged. This is not unlike a stroke, except in a stroke, the block-age is in the brain itself. Regardless of the cause, the brain's being deprived of oxygen can result in severe damage in mere minutes. Therefore, unless there is a clear directive to withhold such treat-ment, such as a written POLST/MOLST order or, in a hospi-tal setting, a written DNR/DNI order, the usual procedure is to immediately attempt to resuscitate the person. You do not want to waste precious minutes determining what to do, which could directly decrease the chance of recovery.

THE LUNGS AND INTUBATION

For a person found to be not breathing, mouth-to-mouth resusci-tation can be started by a bystander. Once paramedics arrive, intu-bation can be performed, which would involve inserting a tube into the mouth and down the throat into the lungs. Ventilation is then provided. Often, the patient requires sedation while on the ventilator, which makes it difficult for him or her to provide consent for other procedures. Additionally, the person is not able to swallow any food or to speak, as the tube is placed between the vocal cords.

PROLONGED NEED FOR INTUBATION

If intubation and mechanical ventilation are required for longer than two weeks, then the tube down the throat is removed, and a small incision is made in the neck so that a tube can be surgically placed through the throat into the lungs; this is called a tracheostomy. With special training, equipment, and time, the person may eventually be able to speak and to swallow some foods.

BRIDGING THERAPY

As mentioned in the case of John, intubation is sometimes offered as a short-term bridging therapy. If you find yourself thinking that perhaps intubation for the short term is something that would work for you, then you need to write your choices down and to inform your agent. By the same token, if intubation is not something you would ever want, then you need to write that down, and empower your agent accordingly. And if endotracheal intubation, as it's called when the tube enters from the mouth, followed by tracheostomy might be something you would entertain, then write that down, and empower your agent.

THE HEART AND CARDIAC DEFIBRILLATION

As the heart needs to deliver oxygenated blood to the brain and other parts of the body, it needs to be pumping in a synchronized and effective manner. As we discussed earlier, in some cases, this can be achieved by delivery of an electric shock. A machine called a cardiac defibrillator can most safely deliver this electric shock.

Portable cardiac defibrillators are available in healthcare facilities, and "smarter" versions are available on planes and in commercial buildings. This smarter version is known as an automatic external defibrillator (AED), as we discussed briefly earlier.

The AED is smarter because it has built-in technology so that the machine, once placed on a person's chest, can analyze the heart rhythm and determine whether it should intervene by delivering an electric shock to attempt to return the heart to a normal rhythm. Proper use of an AED can be taught to just about anyone. When they first came out, a study showed that grade school students could learn how to properly set up an AED and retain that knowledge.

Defibrillation, when indicated, needs to be done quickly, since just as with the brain, when the cells of the heart are deprived of oxygen, this can decrease the chances of survival. As we say in cardiology, time is myocardium, or heart muscle. This means that with every minute that goes by, the heart is dying cell by cell until it is returned to a perfusable rhythm.

On average, it takes first responders eight to twelve minutes from the time a 911 call is placed to arrive on the scene. Each minute that goes by before the heart is successfully returned to a perfusable rhythm decreases recovery chances by approximately 10 percent.

A public-access AED, one that is available for general use, can possibly decrease the amount of time from that initial call for help to the actual delivery of an electric shock, if indicated. As you walk around, become aware of your surroundings and where the nearest public-access AED is located. Taking a class on how to use an AED and to perform CPR is also a very good idea; you never know when you might need those skills.

SUMMARY

This chapter summarizes standard resuscitation options. There are some experimental treatments, such as cooling the body, that we will discuss later. Also, the next few chapters discuss sustaining options for organs beyond the big three. But the big three are just that: it all starts and ends with airway, breathing, and circulation.

- Oxygen is needed to keep the brain, heart, and lungs functioning.
- If the lungs cannot take in oxygen and use the heart to pump it to the brain and the rest of the body, then survival is seriously threatened.
- Sometimes intubation and mechanical ventilation are offered as bridging therapy. With a tracheostomy, intubation can be provided long term too. Consider under what circumstances you might want these treatment options.
- Consider taking a class in how to use an AED and how to perform CPR.
- Become aware of where AEDs are in places you frequent. Some good examples of locations that are likely to have public-access AEDs available include grocery stores, office buildings, places of worship, libraries, shopping malls, local schools, and airports.
- If you have any further questions, then please contact your healthcare providers and your attorney. Please record your choices, and empower your agent to speak for you in these areas.

5

The Kidneys and Gastrointestinal System: Getting Rid of Waste

The best way to find out what we really need is to get rid of what we don't.

—Marie Kondo

A ROSE BY ANY OTHER NAME WOULD SMELL AS SWEET

After completing the ninth consult form for the new patient who had arrived via air ambulance, the resident was informed that she now held the record for the most consults ordered for one patient in the first twenty-four hours of the patient's stay. She wondered who had the time to keep track of such a thing.

This all started earlier that day, when she got a call from a referring hospital's ER physician. The patient had been standing, waiting for a city bus, when he suddenly had to sit down. A passing police car stopped and offered him a ride to the nearby county hospital. His fiancée accompanied him in the squad car.

Upon arrival to the local ER, he walked in under his own power and conversed with the nurses. Soon, his condition deteriorated right in front of the ER physician. The decision was quickly made to transport him to another hospital for a higher level of care.

Almost immediately after he arrived in the ICU of the receiving hospital, he developed respiratory distress; he was intubated and mechanically ventilated. He developed a high fever, and his heart rhythm became abnormal.

Soon afterward, various family members arrived. His fiancée was at the bedside first. She was soon followed by his adult son, his parents, his two brothers, and the mother of his adult son, who referred to herself as his common-law wife.

The patient's condition deteriorated due to the overwhelming sepsis that was consuming his organ systems. Over the next few days, it became apparent that the antibiotics could not knock out the massive infection. Consulting teams of physicians were lining up to obtain informed consent from the family for a variety of necessary and urgent procedures, including kidney dialysis and extremity amputation.

The various family members and loved ones had different names and nicknames for the patient. Some referred to him as Charles, some called him Charlie, and others knew him as Chuck. The one thing they all agreed upon was that he would not want to live this way, on kidney dialysis and with only one arm. After consulting with legal counsel, all the various family members and loved ones signed the necessary documents to withdraw care. Charles/Charlie/Chuck passed away with his loved ones having come together in support of him, his wishes, and one another.

BEYOND THE BIG THREE

As we discussed in the last chapter, the big three refers to the brain, the heart, and the lungs. In primary resuscitation, this means maintaining airway, breathing, and circulation. These areas must be addressed if there is to be any hope for a meaningful recovery.

Yet beyond these basic areas are other treatments, including hydration, dialysis, nutrition, blood transfusion, and antibiotics. In the next few chapters, we shall address these treatments. I have chosen to discuss them in an organ-focused approach. Let's start with the kidneys and the gastrointestinal system.

KIDNEY FUNCTION

The kidneys are the body's filter system. They process waste and extra fluid from the blood and then push that downstream, to be eliminated as urine. Additionally, the kidneys help to regulate the body's blood pressure, electrolyte balance, and production of red blood cells.

Without sufficient kidney function, the waste will not be filtered and fluid will build up. Electrolytes then go out of normal range, and red blood cells eventually stop being produced. This dysfunction can lead to shortness of breath, edema (swelling), sleepiness or lethargy, and mental confusion.

As the kidney failure worsens, the electrolytes, especially sodium and potassium, can shift out of their normal ranges, which can cause dangerous alterations to the heart rhythm. These heart rhythm abnormalities can cause cardiac arrhythmias, which can lead to the heart stopping.

KIDNEY FUNCTION AND PRESSOR AGENTS

Kidney function can be damaged by persistently low blood pressure, which can result from prolonged time without effective heart function. To help prevent kidney damage, intravenous fluids can be given. If this alone does not elevate blood pressure, then pressor agents (vasoactive medications) can be given. These might help in the short term, but potentially dangerous side effects can result when these agents are required at high doses for a long period of time.

KIDNEY FUNCTION AND DIALYSIS OPTIONS

If the kidneys are not able to function, then there are mechanical options to replace their function. One common option is hemodialysis. Hemodialysis uses a special machine to filter a person's blood to remove waste. Patients with chronic renal or kidney failure, sometimes from diabetes mellitus or long-standing hypertension, may require this treatment up to three times a week on an outpatient basis.

For those patients who develop acute kidney failure, hemodialysis can cause too many changes in their body chemistry and blood pressure. Instead, the same machinery can be used at the bedside to offer a gentler form of kidney dialysis, which is referred to as ultrafiltration or continuous renal replacement therapy (CRRT). Often, as the patient's overall condition improves, the acute kidney failure can resolve without further hemodialysis.

Another type of dialysis is peritoneal dialysis, which uses the lining inside the abdomen to filter waste. This is more effective when the patient can move around and ambulate. Therefore, it is not usually recommended for acute kidney failure, such as would be treated in an ICU setting.

GASTROINTESTINAL SYSTEM AND NUTRITIONAL SUPPORT

Nutrition is necessary for life. The body gets nutrition through the gastrointestinal system. This includes all the parts of the body that take in food, digest it, or break it down. The broken-down food bits then have their energy extracted and absorbed. The remaining waste is expelled. The digestive system starts at the mouth. The gastrointestinal system starts at the stomach and includes the large and small intestines. Most of the breakdown is done in the stomach, and the absorption occurs in the stomach and intestines.

When a patient is not able to swallow food, due to either intubation or an altered mental state that does not allow him or her to swallow effectively, supplemental support can be provided. Nutrition can be provided intravenously for the short term. A more effective way is tube feeding. In the acute phase, this is accomplished by placing a tube through the nose and advancing it into the stomach.

The nasogastric tube can be irritating to the lining of the nose and is not a viable option for the long term. If a longer-term solution is needed, then a tube can be surgically placed via an incision in the abdomen and advanced into either the stomach or the first part of the intestines. The placement of the tube usually depends on the risk of aspiration, which is when feedings come up and go into the lungs.

If the patient is alert, then the tube can go into the stomach. If the patient is in a minimally conscious or persistent vegetative state, then placing the tube past the stomach can lower the risk of aspiration. However, the ability to absorb nutrients can be less with this placement.

In a patient nearing the end of life, the use of artificial nutrition and hydration (ANH) has not been shown to be of benefit. In fact, some studies show that ANH can lead to complications. In an end-of-life situation, it is best to consult with the healthcare providers to determine the best course of action, given your goals and wishes.

SUMMARY

- The kidneys are the filters of excess water and waste from the blood.
- When they are not functioning, many problems can result, including cardiac arrhythmia and death.
- Kidney failure can be treated mechanically, including by hemodialysis, ultrafiltration, or peritoneal dialysis.
- Nutrition is necessary for life. If a person cannot obtain nutrition by eating food by swallowing, then nutrition can be provided by tube feedings.
- Please consult with your healthcare providers to determine what your options might be. Then be certain to write down your choices and to share them with your agent.

6

Blood, Skin, and the Immune System: Keeping Up Our Defenses

Build up your weaknesses until they become your strong points.

—KNUTE ROCKNE

STRONG POINTS IN THE MAKING

I remember how my biochemistry professor in medical school described the skin's roles. The skin is the first defense from germs, and it keeps all the important stuff inside, she was fond of saying. Nowhere in medicine is this better illustrated than in the patient who has been burned.

In burn patients, loss of the protective skin means that the important stuff is no longer inside, but outside, exposed to the elements, so to speak. Additionally, the defensive layers against bacteria and other pathogens have been lost. The severity of this loss is the key to determining the best management of these patients.

To estimate the severity of the burn and the optimal treatment, healthcare providers can use a few methods. The "rule of nines" was developed in the 1940s and is still used to estimate the severity of a burn. This method assigns percentages to large body parts, such as 9 percent for one entire arm and 18 percent for one entire leg. If half of a leg sustained burns, then approximately 9 percent would be attributed to that area. By adding up the areas, the total percentage would be used to calculate fluid-replacement needs, as tissues can dry out without the protective skin layers to keep moisture in. Other methods are also used for children and for obese individuals to more accurately assess the severity of the total burns.

Depending on the severity and percentage of burns present, healthcare providers can better determine fluid-replacement needs, skin grafting, and survival rates.

In this chapter, we will look at three areas that need to be addressed when dealing with a life-limiting illness. They are skin, bleeding disorders, and infections.

SKIN

Even for nonburn patients, the skin is an important defense. A patient who has limited mobility is prone to pressure sores, which can lead to pressure ulcers. The constant pressure to the skin can cause it to break down, and then infections can set up shop in the wound. To combat this, patients require more intense nursing care and frequent repositioning in bed. Specialized mattresses and bed frames can also assist in decreasing constant pressure points.

BLOOD AND CLOTTING ISSUES

Blood is critical for any patient's well-being. Some patients, such as those who are immobilized in bed due to their injuries, can develop blood clots due to inactivity. Also, patients with cancer are at an increased risk of forming blood clots due to a side effect of cancer.

Medicines can be prescribed to help prevent clots. Some patients do not want to take these medicines, preferring that if a blood clot occurs, it is not treated, even if it means their death.

This is an area of treatment that should be addressed with your healthcare provider to understand your treatment goals and so that you understand what he or she thinks is best, given your goals and wishes. Then be certain to empower your agent.

BLOOD AND BLEEDING ISSUES

Also critical to a patient's survival is the presence of oxygenated blood from the lungs to carry the oxygen to the rest of the body. In some cases, such as a severe bleed from a wound or an ulcer, the remaining blood may not be able to carry enough oxygen to supply the body. In those cases, a transfusion of whole blood would be ordered. In other cases, due to the underlying illness, the platelets may not be functioning properly. Treatment for this would be a transfusion of platelets.

If someone were to require a transfusion of blood products, then a plan would need to be discussed. This plan would be between the patient, if able, or the healthcare agent, if appointed, and the healthcare providers. The discussion would center on the risks versus the benefits of the transfusion and would focus on the patient's understanding of his or her disease process and the available treatment goals.

In terms of bleeding, the question would be under what circumstances a blood transfusion would be acceptable. Some people refuse blood transfusions for religious reasons. It is best to discuss these potential scenarios and options with your healthcare provider, and then empower your agent regarding your preferences.

THE IMMUNE SYSTEM AND ANTIBIOTICS

Another aspect of therapy would be the use of antibiotics. In some cases, such as our earlier story of John, a patient can present with a bacterial or fungal infection that can be successfully treated, and the patient can be released from the hospital.

In other cases, a patient can develop an infection while in the hospital for other issues. In this case, the infection is considered iatrogenic, or hospital-acquired. These infections can develop because of a weakened immune system in an already ill patient. In some cases, these infections are very hard to treat successfully.

One of the most common infections is pneumonia, which is an infection in the lungs. Pneumonia is the most common cause of all hospital admissions, second only to childbirth. It also is a common cause of death in elderly persons, despite advances in antibiotic therapy.

SUMMARY

- In this chapter, we reviewed three body systems that help patients stay healthy: the skin, the blood, and the immune system.
- The skin acts as a barrier, keeping out infections and keeping in fluids.
- Blood carries oxygen to the body. Without enough oxygen, a patient will not survive.
- Abnormal clotting of blood can occur when patients are immobilized in bed. Patients with cancer also often develop blood clots. If these clots travel to the lung or the brain, then they can be fatal.
- The immune system helps our bodies fight off infection. As we age, the immune system does not work as well, resulting in an increased risk of infections. Pneumonia is a common infection that results in hospitalization and can cause death.

Research and Surgery

Primum non nocere. (First, do no harm.)

—Thomas Sydenham

TRAUMA CALL

The line in the hospital cafeteria was particularly long that evening. Not that any of the food was that great, but it was warm and edible. It would do. Being on trauma call was exhausting. The old surgical axiom that starts with "eat when you can, sleep when you can" was so true.

Just as a seat became available in the dining area, the overhead paging system called out, "Trauma code B, trauma code B." That meant a trauma patient was coming in. The "code B" designation identified that the patient was not in good shape. So much for dinner.

When a trauma patient is identified, the clock starts ticking on what we refer to as the golden hour. The initial assessment of the patient and treatment decisions made in those first sixty minutes from the time of the accident are critical to the patient's chances for survival. We start with the ABCs of airway, breathing, and circulation and go from there.

That night, it seemed to have been a one-car crash. The patient was found as the restrained driver. Both her lap belt and her shoulder belt were still on her. However, the front windshield was cracked in a pattern referred to as spidering.

In spidering, there is a center area of damage to the windshield that corresponds to the area of impact. This is often from the person's forehead. Out from the center in almost concentric circles are waves of cracking. To some, the cracking pattern resembles a spider's web. This pattern was more commonly seen prior to the advent of airbags in cars.

The patient was noted to be bleeding. Her blood pressure was dangerously low, due in large part to the active bleeding. The paramedics on the scene were concerned that she needed more than just intravenous fluids to support her blood pressure until the source of the bleeding could be identified and treated.

The paramedics searched the patient's wrists for a blue bracelet, which would identify her as having opted out of an active research study on the experimental use of a blood substitute. After seeing no blue bracelet, the paramedics had been instructed to enroll her in the study. The patient was randomized in the field to receive either the study drug or intravenous saline, the current state of care. The patient was then transported to the local hospital for further care.

EMERGENCY RESEARCH CONSENT WAIVER
The state in which the car crash occurred had a medical center that was participating in a clinical trial on the safety and efficacy of a blood-substitute product. People who lived in the state had been notified prior to the start of the study and were given a phone number to call to order a blue bracelet. Wearing the bracelet would alert emergency medical service responders that the person had opted out of the trial. Not wearing the blue bracelet meant that the person had not opted out and therefore had consented to participate in the trial.

Permission for this study was based on Title 21, Section 50.24, Subpart B of the Food and Drug Administration (FDA) Code of

Federal Regulations. This section addresses informed consent requirements for emergency research. Trials of this nature, justified under the FDA Code of Federal Regulations, had been done previously. One good example goes back to our discussion of AEDs. The clinical trial that supported their use had a similar scenario for paramedics to proceed with the trial prior to a patient's hospital admission.

The blood-substitute trial took place at thirty-two medical centers in nineteen states from July 2006 to May 2007. The prehospital scenario as described earlier was straightforward and generally accepted: a person is found unresponsive with life-threatening bleeding, and seeing no blue bracelet as a sign of the person's prior decision to opt out of the trial, paramedics randomize him or her into the trial and render treatment. In the end, the FDA did not approve this drug.

But the FDA and the Department of Health and Human Services (DHHS) can enact emergency research waiver protocols when an appropriate treatment option is identified for a clinical trial. These regulations allow for informed consent to be waived prior to treatment in some emergency research protocols.

INFORMED CONSENT

The issue of informed consent is a major part of why it is so critical to name a durable power of attorney for health care. If a care facility wants to administer a treatment or procedure, then it is required to ask permission prior to proceeding (except as noted earlier). In asking for permission, the facility is required to explain the procedure, including any potential risks and benefits. In that way, you are informed and can decide if you want to proceed or not.

If you are not able to speak for yourself, then your durable power of attorney for healthcare decisions will be asked to give consent. If there is no such agent, then your legal next of kin will be asked. If no legal next of kin can be found, then a court can appoint a guardian to make decisions for you if you are deemed not capable.

A current "hot" area of research is looking at potential benefits from targeted cooling of the body. Therapeutic hypothermia, as it's called, has been studied on cardiac arrest survivors in Europe and Australia. The data show some possible benefit from the procedure, which involves cooling the body for twenty-four hours after a person's heart is restarted after stopping, as in a cardiac arrest.

This research is currently being performed in the United States under the Emergency Release Waiver (ERW). People eligible for this treatment are not in any position to give their own informed consent. In some of the medical centers, a Code Chill announcement is made, which alerts the treatment team of the arrival of a patient who fulfills the requirements for the study.

The basis for this research is based on observations that can be traced back to our prior discussion of drowning victims from the Seine River in the 1700s. It has been noted for years that drowning victims pulled out of colder water did better than when the water temperature was warmer. The question this research seeks to answer is if cooling the body reduces the amount of brain damage after the heart is successfully restarted.

SURGERY

Besides the saying in surgery about eating when you can, there is another adage that all medical students learn: A chance to cut is a chance to cure. In other words, with surgical removal and repair, the patient will survive.

Historically, we believe one of the first surgical procedures ever performed was trephination, creating a hole in the skull. Skeletal remains show evidence that many patients survived this procedure. Whether it cured their disease is unknown.

With the advent of war, battlefield surgeries became necessary. These procedures included amputation and removal of foreign bodies. The foreign bodies changed from arrowheads and darts to bullets as weaponry evolved.

As surgical techniques evolved, curing was not always the primary reason for the procedure. In many cases, the best that could be expected was relief of pain, at least for a short time. Advances in anesthesia helped make surgical procedures more tolerable, and therefore, they were more commonly performed.

An example of a curative surgery would be surgical removal of an appendix. Removal of an inflamed appendix might cure the patient of appendicitis, with the help of antibiotics. In a similar fashion, a tonsillectomy, the removal of enlarged tonsils, might greatly decrease the frequency of throat infections.

However, many other surgical procedures were first developed for pain control and were not thought to be curative. A good example of this is coronary artery bypass grafting (CABG). In this surgery, blood cells trying to flow through blocked arteries in the heart are detoured with a new path in order to relieve chest pain or angina. It does not cure the patient of heart disease. The blocked native arteries are still there. But CABG surgery provides a new, unobstructed path for the blood to travel, thereby relieving pain.

Additionally, in the world of cancer, surgery is a great option to remove cancerous tumors where possible. It is not usually a cure in and of itself. With additional therapies such as radiation and chemotherapy when indicated, there is a greater likelihood of getting rid of the cancerous cells.

SUMMARY

- Clinical trials help us to better determine the best approach to a medical problem. Often, this involves a new medication or device.

- To be eligible to participate in a clinical trial, informed consent is usually necessary.
- If you are not able to speak for yourself, then your agent may be asked to provide consent on your behalf.
- In some cases, an ERW protocol may be enacted. In an emergency setting, you may need to have opted out ahead of time if you do not wish to become a research participant in a clinical trial. Be aware of possible ERW protocols in your area and in areas where you may travel.
- Surgical procedures to either cure a condition or alleviate pain may be offered to you.
- As always, discuss your options with your healthcare providers, and determine your wishes and goals. Also, please write down these wishes and share them with your agent, healthcare providers, and attorney.

Section 3: End-of-Life Care: Palliative and Hospice Services

We live in a very particularly death denying society. We isolate both the dying and the very old, and it serves a purpose. They are reminders of our own mortality.

—Elisabeth Kübler-Ross

DEATH AND DYING

I know that I should not play favorites, but here goes. My absolute favorite uncle, who was also my godfather, was diagnosed with a terminal illness when I was eleven years old. I was devastated. My father brought home a book, *On Death and Dying*, by a friend of his, Dr. Elisabeth Kübler-Ross. In this book, Dr. Kübler-Ross discusses the stages that are necessary components of accepting a terminal illness: denial, anger, bargaining, depression, and acceptance. Although I was not the one with the diagnosis, I needed to travel through those stages myself in order to ultimately accept my uncle's illness. It was a great book then, and it still is. I encourage my clients and their loved ones to read it.

LIVING BEFORE DYING

Hospice (and *hospital*) comes from the same root as the word *hospitality*. A hospice was originally a place for travelers to seek rest and care. The first hospice to care for the dying, while also providing an opportunity to enjoy life with such activities as gardening, painting, and hairdressing, opened in London in 1967 by Dame Cicely Saunders, a nurse, social worker, and physician. Named St. Christopher's after the Catholic saint, who is considered the patron saint of travelers, the facility is still in existence today.

Dame Cicely Saunders traveled to the United States in 1963. She was invited to speak to medical students, nurses, and chaplains at Yale University. In 1968, Florence Wald, the dean of the School of Nursing at Yale, traveled to London to learn more about hospice care. In 1974, taking what she had learned from her time at St. Christopher's, she opened the first hospice in the United States, Connecticut Hospice, which is also still open today.

HOSPICE CARE

Hospice care is a patient-centric, team-oriented approach to caring for patients who are facing life-limiting illnesses or injuries. In addition to excellent medical care, it also addresses pain management, emotional support, and spiritual support. The care is personalized to the patient's values and needs. The patient's loved ones are also included in the care model.

Once it is determined that a patient has a life expectancy of six months or less, he or she is eligible for this transition of care. The primary care providers are the hospice team, with the patient either still at home or within the confines of a hospice facility.

PALLIATIVE CARE

In January 1973, a Canadian surgeon, Dr. Balfour Mount, participated in a discussion group on *On Death and Dying*. As a urology oncologist, he worked with many patients dying from cancer and was shocked to study the conditions in which the patients were dying. In September 1973, he traveled to London to observe first-hand the benefits of St. Christopher's Hospice.

Upon his return to Montreal, he wanted to open a center of care for patients with terminal illnesses. Instead of using the term *hospice*, he coined the term *palliative care* and opened the first palliative care center in North America. Dr. Mount used that term because it is based on the word *palliate*, which means to mitigate the intensity or improve the quality of something.

He saw palliative care as a multidisciplinary approach to offering care to patients who were diagnosed with incurable cancers. Unlike with hospice care, eligibility for palliative care is not based on a presumption of a patient's life expectancy. Palliative care is centered on an understanding that the patient is still actively being treated. Ultimately, it is most likely that the diagnosis, or a complication of it, will contribute to the patient's death. At the point that active treatment is no longer a goal of care for the patient, then transfer to hospice care may be appropriate.

SUMMARY

- Dealing with our own mortality and the mortality of our loved ones is never easy.
- When someone is facing a terminal illness, palliative care can start at the same time as the diagnosis is made. Active treatment aimed at minimizing the disease is a goal of palliative care.
- Once the decision to stop active treatment is made, that is likely the appropriate time to transfer the patient to hospice care.
- Both are team-oriented and patient-focused approaches, with inclusion of loved ones.

- If faced with the diagnosis of a terminal illness, then you might want to ask what palliative care resources are available.
- Additionally, you will want to develop a care plan with your healthcare providers to determine your wishes. As always, please write down these wishes, and share them with your agent, healthcare providers, and attorney.

Pain Management

Find a place inside where there's joy and the joy will burn out the pain.

—Joseph Campbell

THE WORST QUESTION IN MEDICINE

My father retired and moved to be near me. He took great delight in reviewing medical decision making with me or, in other words, quizzing me! When I was on a surgical rotation, he suggested that a monkey could suture a banana skin or an orange peel, but if I really wanted to get good, then I should practice suturing with wet paper toweling, as that was more of a challenge. The hospital operators later shared with me that he would call and identify himself, then ask to be connected to "the young Dr. Pesek." To say that he was proud would probably be a bit of an understatement.

However, as he aged, he developed some health issues. One of the issues was recurring pain in his legs, which robbed him of peace. He often said the nights were the worst. He so wanted to sleep but could not, due to his pain.

Not long after his eightieth birthday, he was hospitalized one last time. I recall being asked what I wanted done. Somewhat tearfully, I replied that the question was not what I wanted done;

that question would lead to a very different answer. The question was what he would want done, and the answer to that was that he would simply want to not be in pain.

JOY COMES IN THE MORNING

The hospital did a great job of managing his pain in the last hours he spent here on Earth. I remember peering out the window of his hospital room. There was a terrible storm outside that night; the only break in the darkness was the lightning. But thanks to the pain medication, he slept. In the morning, he was alert and deferred any pain medication. He turned to me, told me that he loved me, then quietly slipped away. When I next looked out the window, I realized that the storm had passed.

CONTROLLING PAIN

Pain management is a very important aspect of providing medical care. Without pain control, patients can have difficulty getting good-quality, restorative sleep. When dealing with a terminally ill patient, pain control also brings into play a delicate balance. The goal of care for most patients is to provide enough pain medication to adequately remove the sensation of pain. However, there is a concern by healthcare providers that too much pain medication could hasten death.

Let me introduce the philosophical doctrine of double effect. Basically, it means that we understand that giving enough pain medicine to make a patient comfortable could be enough to unintentionally cause breathing to stop. The courts have helped to address this issue. William Rehnquist, the late chief justice of the United States, stated: "It is widely recognized that the provision of pain medication is ethically and professionally acceptable even when the treatment may hasten the patient's death, if the medication is intended to alleviate pain and severe discomfort, not to cause death."

One of the best achievements of our hospice and palliative care centers is mastery of pain management. There are several ways that pain medication can be introduced to the body. Venous access, or using an intravenous line, is usually preferred so that the effect can be easily and quickly controlled. If more is needed, then the rate of infusion into the vein can be titrated up. If less is needed, then it can be titrated down.

SUMMARY

- Pain control is one of the most important aspects of end-of-life care.
- It is important to understand the goals of treatment. Do you want to be aware of your surroundings with a minimal amount of pain medication, realizing that you might feel some pain? Or is your greater concern not being in any pain, and you would rather be medicated so that there is no pain sensation?
- Think about what your goals of treatment would be, write them down, and discuss them with the appropriate people in your life, as you see fit: your agent, your healthcare providers, and your attorney.

Spiritual Support

Yesterday is gone. Tomorrow has not yet come. We only have today. Let us begin.

—Joseph Cardinal Bernardin

COMPETENCE, A SENSE OF HUMOR, FAITH, AND AN INCISION

As a physician, sometimes you feel worn down. So many patients are helped and go on with their lives. For me, it's the ones who died under my care for whom I tend to recall the details of each encounter. The remembrances are not self-incriminating; I don't feel guilty for what I did or did not do. It is more recalling the details of how the patient presented and how the person's loved ones interacted with him or her. Also, it is how we, the medical team, the nursing team, and the spiritual team, all worked together to try to help the patient and his or her loved ones.

Over the years, I've found myself collecting notes of encouragement or appreciation. I recently came across this letter, from June 1994, from a priest who had dropped everything to administer the sacrament of the sick to a dying patient. After the patient passed away, I called the priest to let him know and to thank him for his time. Here is his response.

Dear Catherine,

Some time ago I gave a retreat to some medical personnel. During one of the evening discussion periods someone asked me what I looked for in someone in the medical profession. I told her, "I look for competency, a sense of humor, faith and an incision." I'm not sure if you have had an incision, but I do sense that you possess the other three qualities.

I very much appreciate your return phone call. The fact that you even thought to make the call speaks volumes to me. Frankly, I cannot remember the last time that someone made such a call.

You have an obvious sense of joy, Catherine. This will serve your patients well. Indeed, they will be most fortunate to have you as their physician.

Again, thanks for taking the time to call. You do it well...very well.

Peace to Your Heart,
James Friedel, OSA

SPIRITUAL SUPPORT

Studies show that at end of life, patients want to feel that they made a successful contribution to society. For many, many years, I have had on my desk a quote attributed to Ralph Waldo Emerson:

To laugh often and much; to win the respect of intelligent people and the affection of children; to earn the appreciation of honest critics and endure the betrayal of false friends; to appreciate beauty; to find the best in others; to leave the world a bit better, whether by a healthy child, a garden patch or a redeemed social condition; to know even one life has breathed easier because you have lived; this is to have succeeded.

When I saw patients, I would often remember those words and ask them how they defined their success. For those who gave examples easily and quickly, I would listen to their descriptions and commit the details to memory, to remind them later, and especially their loved ones, how they had defined their success in life.

For those who were unable to give examples, I would probe a bit further and see if I could find some details. I might also ask supporting team members, including social workers and nurses, for their input. Additionally, the patient's loved ones could be a great source of validation of what the patient meant to them.

It is important to remember the details of our accomplishments. Those memories nourish us mentally in times of great stress. Additionally, visits by ministers of the patient's religion, if he or she has one, can also help to reinforce the patient's belief in his or her success in life and to help prepare for the future.

SUMMARY

- Spiritual support may be a necessary part of the healing process for all of us.
- Feeling that we have succeeded in life helps us to accept the limitations of illness and the approaching end of life.
- Loved ones, care providers, and ministers can all contribute and reinforce the successes of a person's life.
- Determine who you would want to be made aware if you were to be hospitalized. Be certain to include your spiritual supporters and their contact information. Be certain to write down this information, and share it with your agent.

10

Special Requests

There is no love without forgiveness, and there is no forgiveness without love.

—Bryant H. McGill

WHAT CAN WE DO FOR YOU?

A patient had been transferred to a tertiary-care facility after he suffered a massive heart attack. The tests showed that he had severe heart damage. Unfortunately, he was not a candidate for any of the therapies that were available at that time. A temporary measure, a balloon pump, was placed through a small incision in his leg. The end of this device was advanced to work in conjunction with his still-beating heart, expanding to help push out more blood to the body, then deflating to allow more blood into the heart. This pattern of expanding and deflating gave his very weak heart a little more time.

However, the balloon pump could not remain in place indefinitely. Over time, an infection would likely arise. The patient and his family were made aware of the gravity of the situation. The patient was asked what he wanted done for him. He requested that his wife and daughter get something to eat, as they had barely left the hospital since his transfer.

After they left, the patient asked that the attending physician contact his son. It had been several years since they had spoken. The son was reached by telephone. By the time the wife and daughter returned to the bedside, the son and the patient had patched up any resentment they had harbored. The whole family was together at the bedside as the patient passed away the next day.

SPECIAL REQUESTS

If you had the insight to know that you were facing your last few days or hours on Earth, what would you want? Would you want to be at home? Would you prefer not to be at home? Would you have a party? Would you just want to be with a few loved ones? What music, if any, would you want to hear? What else would you want? What scents would you like surrounding you? Would it be your favorite flowers or perfume?

Every situation is different, but often, there are special requests that make the burden of the last days and hours of a person's life easier. For some, it may be a last goodbye with a cherished pet. Others request a meal of favorite foods. Even if they cannot eat the meal themselves, the familiar scent of the foods can provide comfort. For others, it is hearing favorite music or perhaps viewing beloved artwork.

As these examples illustrate, it can be important to try to resolve conflicts with loved ones. Often, it is helpful to have a person not involved in the conflict make the initial contact and update the loved one on the patient's condition. Hopefully, that person will be receptive to meeting. If a face-to-face meeting cannot happen, then consider having the patient dictate a letter to send to the person.

SUMMARY

- If you knew you were going to die in the next few days, what would you want to do now?

- Where do you want to be? Do you want to be in your own home, in your bed? Or would you prefer not to be at home?
- Who do you want to have around you?
- What does the room look like? Is it filled with lively music and lots of friends? Is it just a few loved ones and classical music?
- Is there anyone you would need to reach out to, to resolve a conflict? If that person is not able to meet you face-to-face, then what would you want to write in a letter?
- Please determine your wishes, write them down, and inform your agent.

11

Organ Donation

Love is our true destiny. We do not find the meaning of life by ourselves alone; we find it with another.

—THOMAS MERTON

A GIFT WAS GIVEN

One hot summer day just before nightfall, the ER in a small community hospital was relatively peaceful, save for the fireflies twinkling out front. This peaceful state was shattered by an ambulance siren in the distance and the crackling sound of the radio in the ER.

Paramedics were bringing in a young girl who had been swimming in a nearby lake with a group of friends. The friends lost sight of her and searched for almost an hour before they found her submerged in the water.

As this occurred in the days before cell phones were common, the friends were forced to find help by driving her to a fire station. The paramedics then brought her to the hospital. Unfortunately, she had been without oxygen for a very long time prior to arriving in the ER.

Testing showed that the patient was without brain activity. Her parents were devastated by the news. She was young and had her whole life ahead of her, including plans to graduate from high school the next week and then go to college to study nursing.

As one of her volunteer projects, she had spent time in a nursing home near her home. Her parents knew that she wanted to work with elderly people. Now, in the space of one afternoon, all that was changed forever.

The topic of organ donation was discussed with her parents. Because of her volunteer work, the girl had told her parents that she wanted to be an organ donor. One of the patients in the nursing home was going blind and needed a cornea transplant. According to her parents, this had made quite an impact on her.

The state organ procurement agency was notified. Representatives came and counseled the family. After all the paperwork was completed and the testing was done, the girl's corneas were accepted for transplant.

A few months later, the community hospital received a lovely note. The corneas had been successfully transplanted into an elderly person. Because of that family's generosity in the face of sorrow, the gift of sight was given back.

ORGAN DONATION

Organ donation is a medical procedure where an organ is removed from a donor and implanted in a recipient. The donation of organs after death so that someone's life can be better is a very noble idea. The first organ donation was in 1954, with a living related donor, the twin brother of the recipient. Both survived the operation and had long lives.

While a person is alive, he or she can agree to be an organ donor. In many states, this decision can be made when obtaining a driver's license. In these cases, the license will be marked to alert healthcare providers that the person has agreed to organ donation.

A person can be any age to be an organ donor. A young person's consent can be signed by his or her parents or legal guardians. The oldest organ donor to date was ninety-two years old.

Certain infections or medical conditions may limit the ability to transplant all possible donated organs. Typically, organs that are used for donation include heart, lungs, kidneys, pancreas, liver, intestines, and thymus. Tissue donations can include skin, corneas, heart valves, tendons, and bones.

Organ donation in the United States is organized by state. The care that you receive if you are an organ donor should not differ from the care you receive if you are not an organ donor. The medical team that treats you while you are alive is totally separate from the transplant team. Testing is done to determine which organs and/or tissues may be acceptable for donation. The costs for these tests are not passed on to donor patients or their families.

After the donations are complete, the family may plan for a funeral. Often, the donor organization will write a letter informing the donor family how the organs and/or tissues were used. This can be of great comfort to a family that is grieving the loss of a loved one, as they learn how their loss is helping others to live.

SUMMARY

- Organ donation is a medical procedure that removes organs and/or tissue for implantation into others who are ill and require the donation.
- Patients of all ages can be accepted as organ donors.
- The medical care a potential organ donor receives should not differ from the care someone who does not donate organs receives.
- The gift of organ donation can be a great comfort to a grieving family, knowing that they were able to help another patient and his or her loved ones.

12

Withdrawing Care

*Just living is not enough…one must have sunshine, free-
dom, and a little flower.*

—Hans Christian Andersen

SUNSHINE, FREEDOM, AND A LITTLE FLOWER

The pager vibrated in the pocket of the white coat. A transfer patient was due to arrive in a few minutes. Few details
were known of the patient's condition, other than it was an elderly
female patient who had been intubated locally. A room in the ICU
was made ready for her arrival.

Soon afterward, the patient's son and daughter-in-law arrived.
They shocked the ICU team with their request. They had asked
for the transfer so that the patient's living will could be honored.
The family produced a copy of the living will. It started with the
words: "If a day goes by that I cannot appreciate the warmth of
the sun on my face, or the scent of a blossoming flower, then I
have exceeded my time here on Earth."

The ICU team was at a loss. Patients were normally transferred for a higher level of care, not for removal of care. A "terminal wean," or withdrawal of the ventilator, could certainly be
done, and was done when appropriate, but this seemed early in
the care plan for the treating team.

After a careful examination of the patient, followed by a thorough review of the accompanying paperwork and a call to the transferring physician, it seemed the patient did not have a good prognosis. She was considered terminally ill and would never be able to come off the ventilator due to a severe and debilitating neurological illness without other treatment options. Consultation with the hospital's legal advisers came next. A terminal wean could be done, but it would require two physicians not involved in her care to independently review all the data and to examine her. If they both came to the same conclusion, then the withdrawing of care could begin.

The physicians' findings concurred with what was already evident, and these findings were then documented in the patient's chart. The family members were counseled and asked what they needed. They requested that a tape of Gregorian chants be played. They also requested to remain at the bedside.

All nonessential equipment was removed. The family members were provided with adequate space and seating. The music was started, and the lights were dimmed. The patient was sedated, and the ventilator was turned off. The physician stayed at the bedside to ascertain that both the patient and her family were comfortable. The family chanted along with the music, and the patient's life functions ceased.

Afterward, the family members were invited to stay for as long as they needed. The music continued at their request. As they left the bedside for the final time, they thanked the ICU team for their kindness and offered a copy of the music for other families to use in such a situation.

WITHDRAWING CARE

Withdrawal of care is a misnomer. Care is not being withdrawn. Instead, we should call it withdrawal of life support. When referring to this type of withdrawal, it usually means removing the ventilator that has been forcing air into the patient's lungs.

This withdrawal is not unlike a search for a missing person. Early on, there is great hope for improvement, and the mission is referred to as search and rescue. However, over time, as we look at the whole picture and realize that meaningful improvement is not going to occur, the mission is changed to search and recovery.

When patients are first intubated and mechanical ventilation is started, the goal is to successfully treat them medically and to return them to a state where they can breathe on their own. The ventilator settings are adjusted as needed to provide the minimal amount of support. Some patients can be successfully weaned from the ventilator. For other patients, however, this is not the case.

Once this decision is reached, the patient, if aware, and his or her loved ones should have a meeting with the care team. At this meeting, the facility's protocol for withdrawing life support should be explained. In planning the time of withdrawal of life support, the loved ones should make the care team aware of anyone the patient would want present. Once all the loved ones are available, the care team should make certain to address any questions.

Appropriate pain medication should be given and continued throughout the withdrawal process. Monitoring that is no longer beneficial, such as blood work and chest X-rays, likely will be stopped. Consulting services might stop by to offer their support but likely will not ask to displace loved ones from the room for examination purposes. Nonessential medications may be discontinued.

Often, the curtains around the bed are drawn to give the patient and his or her loved ones as much privacy as possible. Additionally, the lights in the room are usually dimmed. Soft music can often add a touch of comfort and peace to the room. The presence of a minister is often requested.

After the patient has died, a brief examination is necessary to confirm the death. Bereavement counseling is often available for the loved ones. Palliative and hospice care team members will often be available to provide their support.

SUMMARY

- Withdrawal of care is a misnomer. Care is not withdrawn. The healthcare team will still care for the patient.
- A better term might be *withdrawal of life support*. Usually, this involves removing the ventilator, which has been mechanically supporting the movement of air into the patient's lungs.
- This decision is not made lightly. The patient's wishes and the goals of treatment should be well-known to the healthcare team prior to this point.
- Once the decision has been made, a meeting with the patient, if aware, and loved ones should take place. All questions should be answered.
- The timing of the start of withdrawal should be when all the loved ones who wish to be there are at the bedside.
- All nonessential medications and procedures should be discontinued.
- The room should be made as private and comforting as possible. This may include closing curtains and dimming lights.
- After the patient has died, a brief examination may be necessary to confirm the death.
- Bereavement services should be available for the loved ones.

Section 4: Special Needs

Too often we underestimate the power of a touch, a smile, a kind word, a listening ear, an honest compliment, or the smallest act of caring, all of which have the potential to turn a life around.

—Leo Buscaglia

SPECIAL CASES

So far in this book, we have focused mainly on adult patients who are competent to make their own decisions. However, there are some special cases that require a bit more planning. I would like to discuss them briefly in this section:

- Children
- Pregnancy
- Dementia
- Unbefriended patients

Children

Life is a book. The fact that it was a short book doesn't mean it wasn't a good book. It was a very good book.

ATTRIBUTED TO AMOS TVERSKY

IT WAS A VERY GOOD BOOK

The patient was just six weeks short of celebrating her seventy-sixth birthday. She proudly told everyone that when they asked her age as she was being admitted from the ER. Today was her granddaughter's ninth birthday. She had other things to do than be in the hospital, and she let them know that. But first, it had to be determined what was wrong so they could try to make it better.

We have a lot of sayings in medicine. One is "When you hear hoofbeats, think horses, not zebras." It is another way of saying that common things happen commonly. If a person presents in the Midwest in the middle of winter with a cough, then it could be a cold, the flu, or pneumonia. It is not likely to be some obscure tropical disease. I get that.

The only problem with that, for me, is that I grew up near a zoo; I saw and heard zebras almost every day during childhood. Neither the zoo nor anyone I knew had horses. Before I make any assumptions about a patient's diagnosis, perhaps I need to learn some details. Has the person just flown back from some tropical location? If so, then that tropical disease isn't looking quite so obscure now, is it? For me, that saying has always seemed a bit narrow-minded, if not downright backward.

Back to the seventy-five-year-old patient in the ER. She complained of both chest pain and shortness of breath. It turned out she had not one but two major health problems. She had both a heart attack and a blood clot in her lung (two different sets of hoofbeats!). Soon, she had a stent placed in the coronary artery in her heart; an umbrella device was also placed in a major blood vessel so that no more clots could travel to her lungs. This left her with two very good reasons to be given blood thinners.

Her hospital course was smooth. She completed cardiac rehab and did well. Plans were made for her to go home. Finally, the day of discharge arrived. The granddaughters were in the car, eager to see Grannie out of the hospital. They waited downstairs with flowers and balloons. A birthday cake was at home, awaiting Grannie's expert application of the buttercream frosting.

However, Grannie did not do well on blood thinners. It was quite a balancing act to get the doses of the medications correct. Just before she was scheduled to go home, she developed a severe nosebleed. It was bad. Very bad.

The discharge was canceled. The bleeding would not stop. Finally, an ear, nose, and throat (ENT) specialist had to perform a procedure to stop the bleeding. The procedure worked, and the bleeding eventually stopped. But by then, the patient's oxygen levels had started to fall. Ultimately, she required intubation, mechanical ventilation, and blood transfusions. The extra fluid made her already stressed heart and lungs have to work even harder.

Finally, after all the bleeding issues resolved, she just could not come off the ventilator. She had been exposed to some chemicals earlier in her life, and her lung function had been greatly compromised. Her level of activity was such that it had not previously been an issue for her.

At first, she did well on the vent. The granddaughters visited; she hugged them and was so happy to see them again. But over time, the tissue in her throat was sore from the endotracheal tube. She required heavy sedation so that the ventilator would be more comfortable for her to endure. But the level of sedation made weaning her off the vent impossible.

The granddaughters wanted their Grannie back. The family had started looking for a home with a first-floor bedroom and bathroom, so she could move in with them. They were all focused on her recovery and the birthday celebration they would have with her.

The older granddaughter asked that they make it a double celebration, as she had been away at camp and did not get to celebrate her birthday with Grannie. Then she thought a bit more and asked when Grannie's parents had died. When she was told how long it had been, the granddaughter commented that perhaps it was time for Grannie to celebrate with them again soon.

The hospital asked the family what to do. They replied that she would want to undergo a tracheostomy. This was based on prior conversations that they had had with her.

Grannie had undergone elective hip replacement surgery a year earlier. This procedure had motivated her to determine her advanced directives. She had opted for a written durable power of attorney for healthcare decisions with empowerment of her chosen agent. Her agent knew that Grannie's goals and values aligned with wanting to be with her family, if she was mentally alert, which she had been prior to the sedation, and there was no reason to believe that she would not be again. Perhaps, given more time, she could be weaned off the vent and have the tracheostomy removed.

The night before the tracheostomy was to be performed, Grannie suffered a major stroke; the next morning, care was withdrawn. She died one week prior to her seventy-sixth birthday. At her funeral, her granddaughters spoke of the celebration that they imagined was occurring with Grannie's heavenly family. They never did frost that birthday cake, though.

WHEN CHILDREN HAVE A LOVED ONE WHO IS ILL

Children look to their parents for order in their lives. When a loved one is ill, experts recommend having a private discussion that starts with open-ended questions, such as "How do you think Grandma is feeling?" By starting with this question, you can quickly gauge how aware the child is to any changes. Does the loved one look ill? Has she been doing less? What do these changes mean?

When discussing a terminal illness, it is recommended to use concrete terms such as *death* and *dying*. Explain that the illness is no one's fault, especially not theirs.

Help them to realize that death is not like going to sleep. The person is not coming back. But the child's loved one will no longer be in pain, and his or her memories of the person will live on. Help the child pick out a special item or picture that will help him or her remember the deceased loved one.

WHEN CHILDREN ARE ILL

Having a child who is ill can be extremely stressful. On planes, flight attendants remind us during the safety announcements to put on your oxygen mask first, so you can then take care of others. Generally in life, get the support you need to work out your feelings so you can successfully comfort your child.

It would be easy to either become too permissive or to restrict the child's activities. Either extreme is not best for the child. Try to keep up everyone's normal routines as much as possible.

Speak with your child. Ask what he or she is feeling. Is she feeling tired and unable to do as much? Are his classmates treating him differently? Help the child work through possible strategies to handle these situations.

Try to allocate special time with any siblings who are not ill, so they know you love them and have time for them as well. Ask them about their concerns. Help them work through how they can help their ill sibling.

SUMMARY

- The death of a loved one can be very difficult for a child.
- When speaking with children, be certain to be in a comfortable and private spot. Allow them to express their understanding of what is happening and to ask questions.
- Reinforce that the loved one's illness is not their fault.
- Help them understand that death is not going to sleep. The loved one will no longer be with them physically but will no longer be in pain.
- Consider picking out a special item or picture, and allow the child to have it nearby as a reminder of the loved one.
- When the child is the one with the illness, make certain to take care of yourself so you can be of help to him or her.
- Ask the child how he or she is doing and what changes he or she is experiencing. Try to maintain as normal a routine as you can for the child.
- Be certain to make time for the ill child's siblings, so they know they are special and loved as well. Ask them for ideas on how to care for their ill sibling.
- Be certain to reach out to healthcare providers, social workers, psychologists, and psychiatrists as needed for support.

Pregnancy

I am a thousand winds that blow. I am the diamond glint on snow.

—Mary Frye

DIAMONDS GLINT ON THE SNOW

One wintry February day, a mother-to-be told her husband that she had quite a headache. She did not want to take any medicine for her headache for fear that it would harm their unborn child. She instead decided to lie down and take a nap.

Later that day, the husband went to check on his wife. He found her unresponsive and called for help. She was transferred to a hospital. Once she had been evaluated, she was found to be suffering from a previously undiagnosed brain aneurysm. The aneurysm had caused a weak spot in an artery in her brain that caused the blood vessel to burst and bleed, putting pressure on her brain. As the skull encloses the brain, the bleeding had caused permanent damage, leaving her brain dead.

Next, attention was turned to the unborn baby. Tests revealed no abnormality in the baby. The pregnancy was almost far enough along that the baby could survive if born then. But if there was some way to keep the mother intubated and mechanically ventilated, then the baby would have more time for its lungs and the rest of its body to better develop.

The family agreed that the patient would want to remain on life support for the good of the child. The healthcare providers did their best to maintain a healthy environment for the child. For the next few weeks, the loved ones watched over the situation.

Finally, tests showed that the baby's lungs were developed enough. The baby could be born by Caesarean section. The patient's husband was present and saw the miracle of his child's birth.

The baby seemed healthy. Gently, it was placed on its mother's chest for a few minutes of time together. Afterward, the baby was taken to the nursery.

The new father asked for time alone with his wife. When he was ready, the life-supporting machines were silenced. After saying goodbye to his now-dead wife, the father walked to the nursery to take care of his child.

CHALLENGES OF PREGNANCY

As we discussed earlier, in certain states, when a woman is pregnant, a previously written advanced directive could be invalid. I recommend that you consult with your attorney, but you might want to add some language around "in the event of a pregnancy, these still are my wishes." Or readdressing your current advanced directive, with your signature, date, and number of gestational weeks, might be something your attorney advises to show that you have addressed this issue while pregnant.

Another situation where it might be advisable to readdress advanced directives, or complete them if they're not already done, is in the case of an unmarried couple having a child together. If a medical emergency arises rendering the mother-to-be unable to speak for herself, then her partner might not have any right to decide what happens to her. Ideally, the mother-to-be would designate her partner, or some other interested party, as the durable power of attorney for healthcare decisions. Otherwise, medical personnel will turn to the next of kin, which in most states would likely be a member of the woman's family.

SUMMARY

- Having an advanced directive completed and an agent for healthcare decisions designated is especially important during pregnancy.
- If you prepared an advanced directive prior to becoming pregnant, then you might need to reconfirm your choices once you are pregnant.
- If your next of kin is not the person you would want making decisions for you, then you need to designate the person you would want making decisions as your agent for healthcare decisions.
- As always, discuss your beliefs and wishes with your healthcare providers, attorney, and agent. Document in writing both your choices and the timing of those choices in terms of your pregnancy. In some states, your wishes might not be honored when you are pregnant. Consult with your attorney for more information.

15

Dementia

My father always used to say that when you die, if you've got five real friends, then you've had a great life.

—Lee Iacocca

A GREAT LIFE AND A GREAT DEATH

My grandmother had the most beautiful long brown hair I have ever seen. As a child, I would watch her stroke it with a brush and literally make her hair shine. Then she would gather it all up and swirl it on top of her head, using long tortoiseshell hair clips to secure it in place.

As she aged, she developed what was then called hardening of the arteries. When my mother and I visited her, she was confused and would refer to my mother, her daughter, as her long-deceased mother. I was no longer her granddaughter, but instead, in her mind, I was her little sister.

Initially, as her memory worsened, my grandfather was unable to manage with her at their home. She was placed in a care facility. She was unable to brush her own beautiful hair or to set it up in that perfect bun. Instead, someone brushed it for her and placed it in long braids on either side of her face, as if she was indeed the young girl in her confused mind.

Later, with much assistance, she returned to her home with my grandfather. As the end of her life was nearing, the family was summoned. My mother and I approached her bed with hesitation. I prepared myself for what I thought was inevitable. I expected that my grandmother would greet me this last time as if I was my great-aunt.

Instead, Nana seemed to have escaped the clutches of the fog her mind had been in for so long. She sat up and kissed my mother and me, greeting us by our actual names for the first time in many years. Then she turned toward a corner of the room and started speaking in her native Italian.

After a few minutes, she swiftly turned to my mother, gently admonishing her, in English, for not telling her of her brother's death, which had occurred a few years earlier, while she was lost to our time. She then smiled at us, settled back down on her pillows, turned again toward the corner of her bedroom, and breathed her last.

My grandmother was very fortunate to have the kind of death she had wanted, a happy death. She died in her own bed, at home, with loved ones around her, without pain, and very much aware that she was loved.

She had made it clear that this was what she wanted long before her illness fogged her mind. Her family had been able to make this happen for her. It was a great example for me to see how transitioning to the next phase could be.

DEMENTIA

Dementia is an umbrella term for a syndrome of diseases that negatively impact memory, communication, and the performance of daily activities. One of the diseases within this umbrella term is Alzheimer's disease. The diagnosis of Alzheimer's disease can be confirmed after death, by brain biopsy.

Whatever the cause of the dementia, it is critical that the person make his or her choices for end-of-life care known. If this discussion is delayed, then the patient could lose all decision-making capabilities, and any decisions could be left to the patient's next of kin.

As we have discussed previously, clearly stating wishes and goals is so important. Decisions on possible treatments, such as the long-term use of artificial nutrition and hydration, kidney dialysis, antibiotics, or surgical intervention, need to be addressed soon after the diagnosis of dementia is made.

SUMMARY

- Dementia is an umbrella term for a group of diseases that cause loss of memory, communication, and performance of activities of daily living.
- A common disease under the dementia umbrella is Alzheimer's disease.
- Once a diagnosis of dementia has been determined, the patient's wishes and goals of care should be discussed.
- If this conversation is delayed, then the patient could lose the ability to make his or her own healthcare decisions due to the degenerative nature of the disease.
- If the patient is no longer considered competent to make his or her own decisions, then care choices may revert to the next of kin.
- To remain in control of what is done, it is imperative that your choices are known and documented. Please consult with your healthcare providers, attorney, and agent as soon as possible.

16

Unbefriended Patients

The past is behind, learn from it. The future is ahead, prepare for it. The present is here, live it.

—Thomas S. Monson

WHERE'S THE FIRE?

The pager displayed an unfamiliar number. Upon dialing the number, the first mystery was solved. The caller was a physician on duty in the psychiatric unit of the Veterans Administration hospital. The physician had a recently admitted patient with a history of heart disease and wanted him seen by the cardiology service.

The patient was not complaining of chest pain. He had been admitted after calling the local fire department to report a fire earlier that day. Upon arriving at his home, the firefighters could not locate any evidence of a fire. When they asked the patient where the fire was, he pointed to an area right in front of his eyes. In the view of the firefighting experts, this man did not need the fire department, he needed other help.

He was briefly evaluated at a local VA facility. Following that, he was transferred to the regional VA hospital for further care. He still saw fire everywhere he looked.

When asked to describe what he was seeing, he stated that everything he looked at seemed to be surrounded by fire or a yellow halo. He seemed to understand that there was no fire, but he still saw what looked like fire to him. He sounded competent, but what was causing him to see fire?

Upon further questioning, he also admitted to a lack of appetite over the last few weeks. Additionally, he had felt weak and complained of a headache. In reviewing his rather long list of medications, one drug seemed to stand out. The patient was on digitalis.

Digitalis is a drug isolated from a beautiful flowering plant, the foxglove. The first published use of digitalis dates to 1785. It is commonly prescribed to increase the heart's ability to pump effectively.

When taken as prescribed, it can be a very effective medication. If too much digitalis is consumed, then side effects can include a lack of appetite, weakness, and headache. In severe cases, patients report seeing yellow halos around objects.

Once the healthcare providers had a pretty good idea of the source of the fire, tests such as a tracing of the heart's electrical activity, or an electrocardiogram (EKG), and blood work confirmed the diagnosis of digitalis toxicity. With treatment, the patient improved. The yellow halos disappeared too.

Upon further questioning, the patient shared that he had lived with his parents since his honorable discharge from the military. His father had died years earlier, and his mother had died about two months prior to this hospital visit. As an only child and a bit of a loner, he had no friends or family. Due to a misunderstanding, he had confused his medications and was taking the digitalis an extra two times a day.

Once he was stable for discharge from the hospital, the question arose as to where he should go. The local fire department had notified the VA that his home had been inspected and was condemned due to various safety and health issues. The VA social worker worked to find him a new home.

He was found to not have the mental capacity to live on his own. After an extensive search for any family or friends, he was eventually declared "unbefriended." He was then transferred to an old soldiers' home. A fellow vet at the same home later wrote a note on his behalf. He wanted to share how happy he was in his new home. Additionally, he reported that he was eating better and was no longer seeing any fires.

UNBEFRIENDED

The unbefriended patient is someone I hope none of you ever will become. It is a term that is used to refer to a patient who lacks the mental capacity to make decisions for himself or herself regarding his or her own health care and has no identifiable next of kin who could act in his or her best interests as an agent or surrogate decision maker.

In some cases, a court-appointed guardian steps in to act as the unbefriended patient's healthcare agent. However, this guardian may never have previously met the patient. Additionally, the guardian may not truly know the patient's wishes regarding healthcare choices. In short, this is a less-than-ideal situation for anyone involved.

SUMMARY

- *Unbefriended patient* is a term used to refer to a patient who lacks the mental capacity to make decisions for his or her own health care and has no family as next of kin who would act in his or her best interests.
- A court-appointed guardian may need to step in and to act as the patient's healthcare agent.
- In some cases, the guardian does not know what the patient's healthcare choices truly are.

Conclusion

I shall pass this way but once; any good that I can do or any kindness I can show to any human being; let me do it now. Let me not defer nor neglect it, for I shall not pass this way again.

—Etienne de Grellet

April 16 has been designated as National Healthcare Decisions Day. The placement of this event on the day after income taxes are due in the United States is no coincidence. It was inspired by Benjamin Franklin's famous quote from 1789: "In this world nothing can be said to be certain, except death and taxes."

This book has been a labor of love and a few tears. Hopefully it is not a depressing body of work one must trudge through but a frank conversation between you and me, meant to provoke you, to empower you, and to allow you to life the live you want, right up to the end. I believe you want to be in control of your life and your choices. Let's do it, and let's do it well.

May peace be among you!

Acknowledgments

No man is an island, entire of itself; every man is a piece of the continent, a part of the main...Any man's death diminishes me, because I am involved in mankind, and, therefore, never send to know for whom the bell tolls; it tolls for thee.

—DONNE

MERCI BEAUCOUP

This book would not have been possible without the love and support of my family and friends. Thanks especially to my co-madre and co-padre, who lovingly encouraged me and even cared for my children so I could devote time to finishing this book. *Grazie* to my family for allowing me to share our stories, especially of my grandmother. Although Nana was born in the United States, her Italian heritage is a large part of what made her so special to me.

A special thank you also to my husband and children for their patience with this passion of mine. Thank you to all the nursing staff, respiratory therapists, hospital administrators, chaplains, and fellow physicians who every day try to do the right things for their patients. And last, but certainly not least, thank you also to all my clients and their loved ones, who allow me the privilege of being a part of their lives.

A synonym is a word you use when you can't spell the other one.

—BALTASAR GRACIÁN Y MORALES, SJ

NOTES

Chapter 1

1. Richard E. Kerber, Lance B. Becker, Joseph D. Bourland, Richard O. Cummins, Alfred P. Hallstrom, Mary B. Michos, Graham Nichol, et al., "Automatic External Defibrillators for Public Access Defibrillation: Recommendations for Specifying and Reporting Arrhythmia Analysis Algorithm Performance, Incorporating New Waveforms, and Enhancing Safety," *Circulation* 95, no. 6 (1997): 1677–82, https://doi.org/10.1161/01.CIR.95.6.1677.

2. P. M. Dunn, "Perinatal Lessons from the Past: Andreas Vesalius (1514–1564), Padua and the Fetal 'Shunts,'" *Archives of Diseases in Childhood* 88 (2003): F157–F159, doi:10.1136/fn.88.2.F157.

Chapter 2

1. Robert D. McFadden, "Karen Ann Quinlan, 31, Dies; Focus of '76 Right to Die Case," *New York Times,* June 12, 1985, accessed March 13, 2017, http://www.nytimes.com/1985/06/12/nyre-gion/karen-ann-quinlan-31-dies-focus-of-76-right-to-die-case.html?pagewanted=all.

2. Clyde Haberman, "From Private Ordeal to Natural Fight: The Case of Terri Schiavo," *New York Times,* April 20, 2014, accessed March 13, 2017, https://www.nytimes.com/2014/04/21/us/

from-private-ordeal-to-national-fight-the-case-of-terri-schiavo.html.

3. Manny Fernandez, "Texas Woman Is Taken Off Life Support after Order," *New York Times*, January 26, 2014, accessed March 13, 2017, https://www.nytimes.com/2014/01/27/us/texas-hospital-to-end-life-support-for-pregnant-brain-dead-woman.html.

Chapter 3
1. "Elements of a POLST Paradigm Form," National POLST Paradigm, accessed April 17, 2017, http://polst.org/elements-polst-form/.

Chapter 4
1. "Learn about Automated External Defibrillators, American Red Cross, accessed April 25, 2017 http://www.redcross.org/prepare/location/workplace/easy-as-aed

Chapter 5
1. "High Blood Pressure," Renal Unit at the Royal Infirmary of Edinburgh, Scotland, accessed March 20, 2017, http://www.edren.org/pages/edreninfo/blood-pressure-and-kidney-disease.php.

Chapter 6
1. Mehmet Haberal, A. Ebru Sakallioglu Abali, and Hamdi Karakayali, "Fluid Management in Major Burn Injuries," *Indian Journal of Plastic Surgery* 43, Suppl. (2010): S29–S36, doi:10.4103/0970-0358.70715.

Chapter 7
1. "CFR—Code of Federal Regulations Title 21," US Food and Drug Administration, accessed March 20, 2017, http://www.accessdata.fda.gov/scripts/cdrh/cfdocs/cfcfr/CFRSearch.cfm?CFRPart=50.

2. "Safety and Efficacy of PolyHeme® in Hemorrhagic Shock Following Traumatic Injuries Beginning in the Pre-Hospital Setting," US National Institutes of Health, ClinicalTrials.gov, accessed March 20, 2017, https://clinicaltrials.gov/ct2/show/study/NCT00076648?show_locs=Y#locn.

3. Adam Feuerstein, "Northfield, PolyHeme Not Long for This World," *The Street*, March 18, 2009, accessed March 20, 2017, https://www.thestreet.com/story/10473728/1/northfield-polyheme-not-long-for-this-world.html.

4. Sameer S. Apte, "Blood Substitutes—The Polyheme Trials," *McGill Journal of Medicine* 11, no. 1 (2008): 59–65.

5. Alfred P. Hallstrom, Joseph P. Ornato, Myron L. Weisfeldt, Andrew H. Travers, and James Christenson, "Public-Access Defibrillation and Survival after Out-of-Hospital Cardiac Arrest," *The New England Journal of Medicine* 351, no. 7 (2004): 637–46, http://dx.doi.org/10.1056/NEJMoa040566.

6. "PolyHeme—Artificial Blood & Emergency Medicine Research," Indiana University Center for Bioethics, accessed March 20, 2017, https://bioethics.medicine.iu.edu/reference-center/topic-guides/polyheme/.

7. "Sudden Cardiac Arrest Treatment: Therapeutic Hypothermia," Sudden Cardiac Arrest Foundation, accessed March 20, 2017, http://www.sca-aware.org/sudden-cardiac-arrest-treatment#hypothermia.

8. Michael C. Townsend, "Acute Surgical Emergencies in Patients at or Near the End of Life," *The Ochsner Journal* 11, no. 4 (2011): 338–41.

Chapter 8
1. Janice Reynolds, Debra Drew, and Colleen Dunwoody, "American Society for Pain Management Nursing Position Statement: Pain Management at the End of Life," *Pain Management Nursing* 14, no. 3 (2013): 172–75, http://dx.doi. org/10.1016.j.pmn.2013.07.002.

Chapter 9
1. "Treating Mental, Emotional and Spiritual Needs at the End of Life," National Institute on Aging, accessed March 28, 2017, https://www.agingcare.com/articles/end-of-life-emotional-needs-150264.htm.

Chapter 10
1. "End of Life Care," Patient.info, accessed March 28, 2017, https://patient.info/doctor/end-of-life-care-pro.

Chapter 11
1. "Information about Organ, Eye, and Tissue Donation," OrganDonor.gov, accessed March 28, 2017, https://organdonor.gov/index.html.

Chapter 12
1. David Casarett, Jennifer Kapo, and Arthur Caplan, "Appropriate Use of Artificial Nutrition and Hydration—Fundamental Principles and Recommendations," *The New England Journal of Medicine* 353, no. 24 (2005): 2607–12, doi:10.1056/NEJMsb052907.

Chapter 13
1. Grace H. Christ and Adolph E. Christ, "Current Approaches to Helping Children Cope with a Parent's Terminal Illness," *CA: A Cancer Journal for Clinicians* 56, no. 4 (2006): 197–212, doi:10.3322/canjclin.56.4.197.

2. Dori Seccareccia and Andrea Warnick, "When a Parent Is Dying: Helping Parents Explain Death to Their Children," *Canadian Family Physician* 54, no. 23 (2008): 1693–94.

Chapter 14
1. American College of Obstetricians and Gynecologists, "End-of-Life Decision Making, Committee Opinion No. 617," *Obstetrics and Gynecology* 125 (2015): 261–67, doi:10.1097/01. AOG.0000459869.98866.91.

Chapter 15
1. "End of Life Care," Alzheimer's Society, accessed March 20, 2017, https://www.alzheimers.org.uk/info/20046/help_with_ dementia_care/80/end_of_life_care.

Chapter 16
1. Thaddeus Mason Pope and Tanya Sellers, "Legal Briefing: The Unbefriended: Making Healthcare Decisions for Patients without Surrogates (Part 1)," *Journal of Clinical Ethics* 23, no. 1 (2012): 84–96.

GLOSSARY

Acute care facility
Where patients receive short-term treatment for severe injuries or episodes of illness or recover from major surgery, such as a hospital.

Advanced directive
A legal document that allows you to describe the kind of medical care you hope to receive if you are unable to communicate for yourself.

Air ambulance
A specially equipped aircraft, either a helicopter or a fixed-wing plane, used to transport sick or injured patients to a hospital in an emergency.

Algorithm
A stepwise process for solving a problem, often built into and automated by a computer.

Allow natural death (AND)
A medical term referring to an order to allow for a patient's comfort and pain management rather than active life-extending treatment.

Alzheimer's disease
A progressive, degenerative disorder that attacks the brain's nerve cells, resulting in loss of memory, mentation, and language skills and behavioral changes. In 1906, Dr. Alois Alzheimer described a patient with these problems. The diagnosis is confirmed by brain autopsy.

Anesthesia
Medically induced temporary loss of sensation or awareness, used prior to a surgical procedure for pain control.

Antibiotics
Medication used to treat or prevent bacterial infections.

Appendicitis
Inflammation of the appendix, an organ attached to the large intestine.

Articulate
To express yourself fluently and coherently.

Artificial nutrition and hydration (ANH)
A chemically balanced mix of nutrients and fluids, provided as a life-sustaining treatment by tube feedings, either directly into the stomach or the intestine or by venous access.

Aspiration
Accidental inhalation of food or other foreign material into the lungs, usually when the patient is unconscious and unable to protect the airway. This often leads to a severe infection in the lungs.

Automatic external defibrillator (AED)
A lightweight, portable device that analyzes a patient's heart rhythm and can automatically deliver an electric shock in an attempt to return the heart to a perfusable rhythm.

Bacterial infection
An invasion of disease-causing microorganisms that grow and reproduce in the body. This often results in tissue injury and can progress to disease. When the microorganisms are bacterial in nature, antibiotics are often prescribed to try to eliminate the progression of disease.

Balloon pump
See Intra-aortic balloon pump.

Bereavement counseling
Advice and support given to people who have lost a loved one to help them work through their grief.

Biochemistry
The study of chemical processes that occur in the body.

Blood substitute
A substance used to replace blood loss due to bleeding.

Brain aneurysm
A bulging, weak area in the wall of an artery that supplies blood to the brain.

Brain damage
Injury to the brain that impairs its function, often permanently.

Brain dead
The state of irreversible brain damage causing the end of independent respiration, regarded as indicative of death.

Bucking the ventilator
Fighting the respirator; involuntarily resisting positive pressure ventilation in a patient with an endotracheal tube in place.

Caesarean section
A surgical operation for delivering a baby by cutting through the mother's abdomen.

Cardiac arrest
Unexpected loss of heart function, breathing, and consciousness, a medical emergency that, if not treated immediately, can cause death.

Cardiac arrhythmias
A group of conditions in which the heart beats abnormally.

Cardiac rehabilitation (rehab)
A medically supervised program to help improve cardiovascular health for people who have had a heart attack, heart failure, coronary artery bypass grafting, or percutaneous coronary intervention.

Cardiac rhythm
The electrical activity of the heart.

Cardiopulmonary resuscitation (CPR)
An emergency lifesaving procedure of compressing the chest to maintain circulation when the heart has stopped pumping effectively.

Cardiothoracic surgery
The field of medicine involved in the surgical treatment of organs inside the chest, including the heart and lungs.

Chest compressions
Applying pressure to the chest to help blood flow through the heart in an emergent situation.

Circulation
The continuous movement of blood through the heart and blood vessels.

Cognitive
Concerned with the act or process of knowing or perceiving.

Competency
The mental ability to manage one's own affairs.

Consciousness
A state of general wakefulness and responsiveness to surroundings.

Continuous renal replacement therapy (CRRT)
A type of dialysis used to treat seriously ill patients in the ICU who develop acute kidney injury.

Cornea transplant
A surgical procedure to replace a diseased portion of the eye with a donated portion.

Coronary artery bypass grafting (CABG)
A type of surgery that can create new routes around narrowed and blocked coronary arteries, increasing blood flow to the heart muscle.

Coronary stent
A metal mesh tube that is inserted and expanded in a coronary artery to improve blood flow.

Curative
Health care that focuses on active treatment to remove disease.

Defibrillator
A device that delivers an electric shock at a preset voltage to the heart muscle to return the heart to a normal cardiac rate and rhythm.

Dementia
A decline in mental ability severe enough to interfere with daily life.

Department of Health and Human Services
A Cabinet-level department of the US government charged with protecting the health of all Americans.

Deteriorate
To become progressively worse.

Diabetes mellitus
A disease in which the body's ability to produce insulin is impaired, resulting in elevated blood glucose levels.

Diagnosis
Identification of the nature of an illness.

Digitalis
A medication prepared from the foxglove plant that stimulates the heart muscle.

Discharge
To release, as in to discharge from a hospital.

Do not intubate (DNI)
A physician order to not insert a tube to assist a patient's breathing.

Do not resuscitate (DNR)
A physician order to not perform chest compressions or insert a breathing tube.

Double effect
The good and bad effects of an action, compared, according to a principle that seeks to justify the action, if the bad effect, though foreseen, is outweighed by the good effect.

Downtime
Duration of time from cardiac arrest until beginning of cardiac resuscitation or advanced cardiac life support.

Durable power of attorney for health care (DPOA-HC)
A document that allows you to name someone else to make decisions about your health care in case you are not able to make those decisions yourself and the instructions for the person to follow.

Ear, nose, and throat (ENT) physicians
Physicians trained in the medical and surgical management and treatment of diseases and disorders of the head and neck.

Electrolyte
An ion, a substance in the body that regulates the flow of nutrients into and waste products out of cells.

Emergency medical services (EMS)
Treatment and transport of people in crisis health situations that can be life threatening.

Emergency research consent waiver
Ability to conduct research on humans in need of medical therapy without obtaining permission to do so.

Endotracheal intubation
A medical procedure in which a tube is placed into the windpipe through the mouth or nose.

Euthanasia
The act of killing or permitting the death of a hopelessly sick or injured individual.

Extraordinary means
Means of preserving life that cannot be obtained or used without extreme difficulty in terms of pain, expense, or other burdening factors.

Feeding tube
A medical device used to provide nutrition to a patient who cannot obtain nutrition by mouth.

Fetus
A developing baby in the uterus.

Full cardiac arrest
The sudden unexpected loss of heart function, breathing, and consciousness.

Fungal infection
An inflammatory condition caused by a fungus.

Golden hour of trauma
The first sixty minutes from the occurrence of a trauma, during which there is the greatest likelihood that prompt medical treatment will prevent death.

Gregorian chants
Church music sung as a single vocal line in free rhythm and a restricted scale in a style developed for the Medieval Latin liturgy.

Heart
A hollow muscular organ that pumps blood through the circulatory system by rhythmic contraction and dilation.

Heart-lung bypass machine
A device that temporarily takes over the function of the heart and lungs during surgery, maintaining blood circulation and oxygen content.

Hemodialysis
A medical procedure to remove fluid and waste products from the blood and correct electrolyte imbalances.

Hospice care
Supportive care provided to people in the final phase of a terminal illness. Focuses on comfort and quality of life rather than on a cure.

Iatrogenic
Relating to illness caused by medical examination or treatment.

Immune system
The system that protects the body from foreign substances.

Incision
A surgical cut or wound of body tissue.

Institutional Review Board (IRB)
A committee formally designated to approve, monitor, and review biomedical research.

Intensive care unit (ICU)
A department of a hospital where patients who are dangerously ill are kept under constant observation.

Intra-aortic balloon pump (IABP)
A medical device that is inserted into the heart to help it pump more effectively.

Intravenous
Existing or taking place within or administered into a vein.

Intubation
Insertion of a tube into a person's trachea for breathing.

Kidney failure
A medical condition where the body's metabolic waste cannot be filtered from the blood.

Kidneys
Organs in the abdominal cavity that regulate fluid balance and filter out waste products from the blood as urine.

Living will
A written document that allows a patient to give explicit instructions about medical decisions to be administered when he or she is terminally ill or permanently unconscious.

Long-term care facility
A facility that provides rehabilitative, restorative, and/or ongoing skilled nursing care for patients in need of assistance with activities of daily living.

Lungs
Organs in the chest (or thorax) that are the principal parts of the respiratory system where inhaled oxygen is transferred to the blood, and carbon dioxide is removed from the blood and exhaled.

Mechanical ventilation
An artificial way to assist or replace spontaneous breathing.

Minimally conscious state
A disorder of consciousness, with partial preservation of conscious awareness.

Minority age
Under the age of majority, at which time the rights and responsibilities of an adult are bestowed, which is eighteen years of age in most locales.

Mortality rate
The number of deaths in an area or time period or from a specific cause.

Mouth-to-mouth respiration
A method of artificial respiration where a person breathes into an unconscious patient's lungs through the mouth.

Nasogastric tube
A tube inserted into the stomach through the nose.

National Healthcare Decisions Day
The day after income taxes are due, a time to think about who you want to speak for you when you cannot speak for yourself regarding healthcare decisions.

Neurosurgeon
A surgeon who specializes in surgery on the nervous system, especially the brain and spinal cord.

Next of kin
A person's closest living relative or relatives.

Orders for life-sustaining treatment
A medical order for someone with a serious illness near the end of life that directs emergency medical services as to what care the person wants.

Organ donation
The process of surgically removing an organ from one person and placing it in another person.

Palliative care
An approach that improves the quality of care for patients and their families facing problems associated with life-threatening illness.

Paramedic
A person trained to give emergency medical care to people who are seriously ill with the aim of stabilizing them before they are taken to the hospital.

Peritoneal dialysis (PD)
The removal of waste products from the blood by a tube placed into the abdomen when the kidneys are no longer working.

Persistent vegetative state
A condition in which a patient is completely unresponsive to stimuli and displays no sign of higher brain function.

Platelets
Cells that circulate in the blood and prevent bleeding by promoting clotting.

Pneumonia
Inflammation of the lungs caused by a bacterial or viral infection in which the air sacs are not able to function.

Polio
A contagious viral illness that can cause paralysis, difficulty breathing, and death.

Pressor agents
Medicines that constrict small blood vessels, which increases blood pressure.

Prognosis
A medical prediction of the future course of the disease and the chance for recovery.

Psychiatrist
A medical practitioner who specializes in the diagnosis and treatment of mental illness.

Pulmonary embolism (PE)
The sudden blockage of an artery in the lung caused by a blood clot that traveled from elsewhere, often the legs.

Pulmonologist
A physician who specializes in the diagnosis and treatment of conditions and diseases of the respiratory system, especially the lungs.

Readmission
Being admitted to the hospital again after discharge within a specific time, such as thirty days.

Rescinded
Voided, revoked, or canceled.

Sedation
Administration of a drug to produce a sleepy or relaxed state.

Sepsis
The presence of harmful bacteria and their toxins in body tissues, typically through an infection or a wound.

Skin grafting
A surgical operation in which a piece of healthy skin is transplanted to a damaged site on the body.

Spidering of the windshield
Damage to a vehicle's windshield, usually caused by an unrestrained driver or passenger. The damage is usually from the person's head or forehead contacting the windshield. An indication of severe trauma to the person.

Terminal event
An illness or injury of such a serious nature that it causes imminent death.

Terminal weaning
Removal of mechanical ventilator support, with an expectation that the patient will not be able to survive without the support.

Tertiary-care facility
An institution with highly specialized medical care, including the ability to offer advanced, complex, state-of-the art procedures and treatments.

Therapeutic hypothermia
Deliberate reduction of core body temperature in a patient who does not regain consciousness after return of spontaneous circulation following a cardiac arrest, also known as targeted temperature management.

Tonsillectomy
Surgical removal of the tonsils.

Trachea
The windpipe: a large membranous tube reinforced by rings of cartilage, extending from the larynx to the bronchial tubes.

Tracheostomy
Surgical construction of an opening in the trachea for insertion of a tube to facilitate breathing.

Trephination
Surgical procedure in which a circular part of the skull is carved away, leaving a hole in the skull.

Tropical diseases
Infectious diseases that are uniquely seen in humid conditions, such as malaria.

Ultrafiltration
A type of kidney dialysis where excess fluid can be removed.

Unbefriended patient
A person who does not have the capacity to give informed consent for the treatment at hand, has not executed an advanced directive and has no capacity to do so, and has no legally authorized surrogate and no family or friends to assist in the decision-making process.

Vasoactive
Affecting the diameter of blood vessels, therefore affecting blood pressure.

Venous access
Provided when a tube is inserted into a vein to draw blood, to monitor, or to administer medication.

Ventilation
The process of air exchange between the lungs and the ambient air.

Viable
Having attained form and development to be able to survive, as in a fetus being viable outside the womb, usually around twenty-six weeks after conception.

Withdrawal of care
Discontinuation of life-sustaining therapies, such as mechanical ventilation, in a patient expected to die without this support.

Zebra
African wild horse with black-and-white stripes and hoofs.

Made in the USA
Lexington, KY
01 June 2017